Diet Slave No More!

Diet Slave No More!

A FUN LITERARY JOURNEY INTO YOUR SELF

Svetlana Kogan, MD

Disclaimer:
The information presented in this book is meant to be used for general resource purposes only; it is not intended as specific medical advice for any individual and should not substitute medical advice from your doctor. If you have (or think you may have) a medical problem, speak to your doctor about it without delay.

ISBN-13: 9780692753071
ISBN-10: 0692753079

To my beloved children, Rachel and Marc.
You inspire me to be a better person every day.

Contents

Preface

This book has a follow-through companion—a Phone App—called Diet Slave No More! Make sure you read the book first, before proceeding to download the app. The app helps you to execute the steps recommended by the book.

I have spent many years writing this little book. Toward the end of my creative process, a Phone App was born. If I consider this book to be my baby, then the app would be my grandchild. And I do not recommend meeting my grandchild app before getting to know her mother book! Of course, should you want to get to know "the grandma", I currently live and work in New York City. Feel free to communicate via the contact page on my professional website www.dtpdoctors.com.

So, if you really want to reach your target weight naturally and maintain it forever, please be patient and read the book in its entirety before using the app.

With warmest regards,

Svetlana Kogan, MD

CHAPTER 1

Who Am I?

Once upon a time, a blond, blue-eyed emigrant from the former Soviet Union—that's me—graduated from Cornell University and entered Sackler Medical School to become a doctor, one of the most ancient and holiest professions humankind has ever known.

I had always wanted to become a doctor since when I was six years old and hospitalized for a suspected appendicitis. Back then, where I am from, parents were not allowed to stay with their children in the hospital, and very sick kids befriended one another. I made friends with a leukemic boy who was sharing the room with me and eight other kids with completely unrelated illnesses. We listened to my transistor radio and told each other jokes to bide our time. My friend was pale but beautiful, and his golden locks made him look like an angel. One night, there was a lot of commotion, screeching sounds of machines and loud voices, and in the morning, my friend's bed was empty. He was "gone," the nurse told me dryly.

The boy's passing had left me choking with tears and an overwhelming desire to do something to avenge his death when I grew up. And what better profession was there to fight sickness than being a doctor? And so, when it was time to choose a career, my path was predetermined. Despite my love for art history and languages, I headed for medical school, driven by my childhood memories and the promises I made.

Medical school was an exhausting but fascinating journey inside the human body. I was extremely lucky to be taught by some of the brightest medical minds of our time. The academics required tons of dissections and memorizations of Latin names and facts. That's where my linguistic gifts came in very handy. Our anatomy professor, Dr. Yoel Rak, was a world-famous archaeologist, who had discovered the oldest human skull on the planet. He tried to infuse the otherwise-dry anatomy material with some refreshing evolutionary points of view. Another stellar researcher, Professor Laron, who had discovered nothing less than a syndrome of dwarfism, was trying to lighten up otherwise mundane endocrinology, the science of hormones.

But my most memorable days of medical school were not spent in the classrooms, of course, but in clinical rotations at the hospitals. This was the real deal. My surgical preceptors were war veterans, and they were tough as nails. They taught me how to think fast under pressure and get things done with the minimum of help and resources available. I would often scrub in with trauma surgeons for the late-night cases. One day, around 3:00 a.m., I was very exhausted and ready to call it a night. It was then that an eighteen-year-old boy was brought into our operating room. He was a victim of a car accident; he had flown forward from the backseat into the windshield of the car. The boy was unconscious and rapidly losing blood pressure. A huge incision was immediately made all the way from his solar plexus to the pelvis by the on-call trauma surgeon, who then launched a hunt for the source of bleeding, which if not stopped would've destroyed this boy's life in minutes. Without any CT scans, the source of bleeding was found swiftly through sheer manual search. It was one of the worst kinds, and once exposed, the depressurized blood burst out at us like a wave. After clamping down all the visibly oozing vessels, the surgeon decided to wash the entire content of the abdomen and to look for other squashed or destroyed organs, which had to be removed. Before the aorta—the largest blood vessel in the body—was clamped, he asked me to feel it, and as I unwillingly placed my fingers on it, I felt this boy's pulsing life. It was very rapid and bounding, and it made me sick to my stomach. The surgeon picked up the boy's intestines and handed them over to me. "Hold on tight," he uttered firmly. "I am going to clean up this mess."

I gasped, as I felt overwhelmed under the weight of the warm and gooey flesh in my arms. All of a sudden, the surrealism of this situation dawned on me: it was 3:00 a.m., I was exhausted, the Yom Kippur War–veteran surgeon next to me was taking out the crushed left kidney, and I was barely standing there, dizzy and tired, ready to collapse, with my arms full of an eighteen-year-old boy's guts. I sensed a noise in my ears and a familiar feeling of flying into the tunnel, the classical vasovagal episode commonly known as "passing out" after prolonged standing in one spot. *To hell with everything*, one of the inner voices in my brain was screaming. *I am gonna lay you down right now.* The other subconscious voice, however, was of a different opinion. It had sent a sharply felt realization down my spine that, by collapsing onto the floor, I would be taking this boy's life by degutting him.

I don't know what force kept me on my feet that night, but I stood there until it was all over. The moment I stepped out of the OR, I collapsed onto the floor in the cafeteria. In the morning I was checking to see if the boy had survived, and to my joy, I discovered him smiling in his bed: "Good morning, Doctor Kogan. I heard you guys worked hard to save me last night."

"I am not a doctor yet," I mumbled, almost choking on the intense feeling that came all over me. I knew I had avenged the death of my childhood hospital friend.

Moments like these made all the sleepless nights worth it—like the first night of my obstetric rotation in Labor and Delivery. I was chasing an Ethiopian woman down the hallway. She had abandoned her bed and stood in the corner, shaking with fear. Back where she was from, babies were delivered only standing up. Delivering her baby in this unusual-for-me position taught me that, in some parts of the world, people prefer to do it this way. Great.

The second night in my new psychiatric rotation, I was held at gunpoint by a psychotic soldier. He demanded to be injected with a sedative, and having received what he wanted, he happily slumped onto the floor. Marveling at the way the events of that day played out, I got lost on my way home from Ichilov Hospital in Tel Aviv. It was a very long walk in the pitch-black, and all I remembered was a cue that I lived close to the museum of Israel. Lucky for me, I came upon a bonfire with a bunch of young people sitting around it and smoking pot.

"Looks like you are lost," they said. Tired and exhausted, I wanted to ask them, "Where is the museum of Israel?" But what came out of my mouth in broken Hebrew at that moment was this: "I am looking for the land of Israel." They all hopped to their feet and started bowing to me, laughing hysterically, and said, "You have arrived!"

Time has a tendency to fly, and before I knew it, my four years were up, and I was graduating from medical school. I was a proud bearer of the Hippocratic oath, had all the empathy in the world, and was ready to never sleep and to always be ready to help my patients.

My internal medicine residency at the New York City's Lenox Hill Hospital has been extremely rewarding and intense. All of a sudden, I was not a student anymore—I was a medical intern. The nurses were paging me for orders, and patient's families were awaiting my care. There was no place for hesitation or doubts. The stress was huge. Back in those days, there was no cap on how long the residents could stay up working, and I often worked eighty-five to ninety-five hours per week.

Two months into my internship, I was walking the hallways of the hospital on my night duty, around 4:00 a.m., ready to "call it a night," which really meant retiring into the stinky, tiny room where I would try to close my eyes on the bed until someone else would page me for something to do. I had finished my rounds, and all the patients I was covering were tucked in. But one patient kept popping up in my mind: an elderly lady whom I had admitted earlier that night with diagnosis of dizziness. I felt an overwhelming "itch" to check up on her one more time, and my legs literally turned by themselves and led me into the room where a feeble old lady was sitting on the floor, clutching her hand to her chest and breathing heavily. Her eyes were closed. She was unconscious. Lucky for Edith (this was her name), I had instantly recognized the signs of pulmonary edema, a lethal condition when untreated, and swiftly took care of it with my textbook-protocol-IV treatments and oxygen.

When she opened her eyes, the first thing she saw was me standing above her. Smiling with deep relief—we came very close to losing this woman on my night watch—I went home to sleep in the morning, and when I came back in seven hours, Edith had already been moved to a regular floor as she felt much better. I was told that she was looking for her "angel with a Russian name." She probably convinced one of the nurses to give her my home address. Little did I know that the feeble old patient of mine was a renowned artist and still painting, despite being in her eighties. Several weeks later I received a package from patient Edith Meisl-Bernhard, which I opened with trembling hands, not knowing what to expect. It was a painting of me as seen by Edith awakening from her unconscious state. I was pondering for weeks about what led me into her room that night…

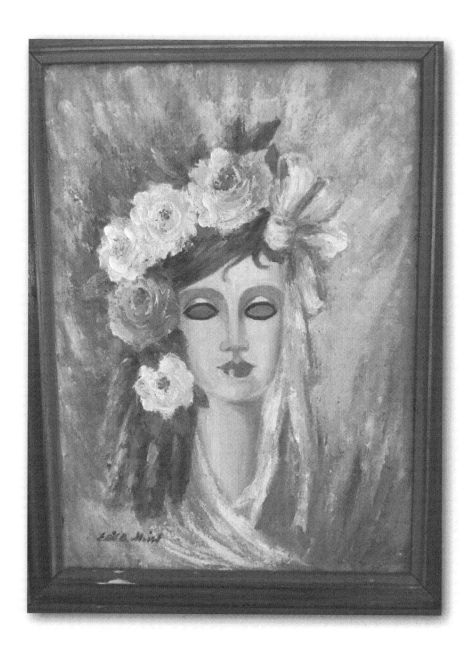

My days as a medical resident were like an emotional roller coaster: some patients were admitted for simple problems, but some never made it out of the hospital. One young woman had refused to abort her dead fetus and, as a consequence, wound up developing an unstoppable bleeding from all the orifices in her body. As a senior resident, I was leading the team of doctors and nurses trying to resuscitate this poor woman for hours. Twenty weeks pregnant myself, I just could not allow myself to let her go. Bags of blood, plasma, and platelets were going into her body and bleeding right out. Intravenous medications were being pushed, and chest compressions would not cease. I had not even noticed that we were an hour and a half past the usual "allowance" for pronouncing someone dead, when they cannot be resuscitated. One of the nurses gently put her arms around me and pulled me away from the bloodbath, saying, "You just have to let go. She is gone."

That night, doubled over on a little bunk bed in my ICU on-call room, I was choking from tears of inadequacy and hopelessness. I was grieving and wailing so deeply that it was surprising I did not have a miscarriage myself. I had learned that I could not save everyone.

Five months later, after what seemed like a sleepless mixture of drama, horror movie, comedy, and tragedy, the residency experience was finally over.

One day before my due date, I was heading over to my two-day board certification exam. I had a car waiting for me outside in case the baby would insist on coming out pronto. The exam proctors were giving me hateful looks—I was a pregnant menace to their peace and quiet. During the exam contractions came and went, and I kept running to the bathroom, accompanied by the outraged exam proctor, but some invisible force had pulled me through these two days of board exams. The day after the board exams, I found myself on the delivery floor of my hospital; only this time I was the patient.

My delivery was bad. Everything that could go wrong went wrong. After twenty hours of breathless pushing, with an oxygen mask on my face, I was wheeled into the operating room and laid onto the bed, where that poor lady patient whom I was telling you about on the previous page had perished twenty weeks before. Doctors and nurses were running around screaming. Forceps, a vacuum device, and curses were flying in the air—but I was calm. I thought that this was my end. Right there. Right where my patient passed away. I could not save her, and it just made sense for me to die right there. Strangely, I was accepting whatever was coming. But something or someone really wanted my baby and me to live on that day, and we miraculously pulled through.

I even survived the forgotten pieces of placenta, which bled out of me the next day, and the kidney infection that followed. I left the hospital quietly, with a catheter in my lifeless bladder and a bag of urine tied to my leg. No matter; I was thrilled to be alive and have my baby. I knew that I was a survivor, and that meant that I had a mission on this earth.

Eventually, my bladder started functioning again, and I was ready for living out my mission. All the knowledge and experience that were overflowing inside of me had to be expressed and shared. I called up the management in my apartment building and asked them if they had a small office to rent. They said that there was a one-bedroom apartment that had been rented out by a now-retired surgeon. Perhaps, I would want to convert that into a primary-care office. I scratched my head: Convert? That would involve the construction people, right?

Someone recommended an inexpensive guy from Brooklyn. He had never done medical offices, but who cares about a resume when you hardly have any money to spend? "So, what are we doing?" he asked, toothpick in his mouth, standing in the center of an old kitchen that was to become my first office.

"Well for starters, let's take down all the walls and build a reception area right here by the door. We'll figure it out from there." He shrugged and went to work on my office-to-be with his two-men crew. I had no one to consult on the layout or design. There were no doctors in my family, and no one in my graduating residency class was opening his or her own office. The odds of new business failure were too high—statistically 95 percent. But when you are driven, nothing matters. I had randomly picked a medical-equipment guy from the yellow pages and invited him into my "office under construction."

It was a beautiful January afternoon when this seventy-five-year-old guy named Norman Schor walked into my office-to-be and froze in his feet. "What is this?" he asked, wide-eyed, referring to the overly high countertop in the reception. "How am I supposed to reach this? Never mind leaning on this to write something down. And what the hell is this?" He was eyeballing the entrance door that was swinging open into the office, straight into him standing at the counter. "This thing is going to nail me dead to the countertop. Who built this?" Frustrated, I conveyed Norman's concerns to my construction guys and asked them to lower the countertop and change the direction the door was swinging. My request must have had devastating effects on their ego, because they decided to just—leave. And they left with almost all of my money that I had paid them forward. To highlight how pissed off they were at my critique, they spilled liquid glue on my floor while leaving.

"In good riddance," I was muttering to myself, as my family and I were scrubbing the floor for two days with a razor blade, cleaning the glue off the new Home Depot tiles.

Norman was my kind angel. He said, "This is not the end of the world, Doc. I will bring in two new construction people and negotiate a decent price for you." He also advised me on the legal requirements for the exam-room size and helped to pick the spots for all the electric outlets and the air conditioner. Thanks to Norman's kind suggestions and my renewed hope and zest, the office construction was finally completed in several months.

On the first day of spring, I announced the opening of the office to the doorman of my building and proudly walked inside my fresh paint–smelling office, wearing a crisp new white coat. Finally, a real doctor! In my own office! My first and only employee, a lady receptionist, gave me an encouraging nod, as I walked into my own consultation room and sank into the furniture from Staples, which I had finished putting together the day before, bolt by bolt. I proudly looked at the diplomas displayed on the walls. The red mahogany of the frames left me satisfied. And so I sat in my plush vinyl armchair—all day. No one came in except the mailman. The same happened the next day—and the next. The phone was silent, and there were no patients in sight. People were not lining up to experience my valuable and fresh knowledge and care. Gradually, restlessness and panic started creeping into my head. I had never felt this way before.

On the one hand, I was overfilled with emotions of empathy for the sick and wanted to share my experience and enthusiasm with the patients. On the other hand, there were no patients to take care of. And what was there, really? A newly built office with all the accompanying expenses and leased-equipment bills, the university and medical-school loans of astronomical sizes that had to be paid off, and the malpractice insurance and babysitting expenses so that someone could stay with my six-month-old child while I was at work.

I was thirty years old and had been in school for twenty-four out of those thirty years. But no school and no one had ever prepared me for the feeling I was experiencing right then—the state that I was in. How was I supposed to act? What was I supposed to do to resolve my situation?

At night, I could not fall asleep, my mind racing in a circular thought of "what do I do?" By morning, I was getting out of bed with a sense of doom and felt really fearful of what the new day was going to bring. I felt hopeless...

Today, rewinding my life's "movie" backward, I am grateful to my fate for starting me off in my professional career by throwing me down low and deep. If it wasn't for having to think day and night about finding my way out of the maze that I was in, I don't think I could ever evolve to become a real healer of the sick: the doctor who not only knows how to treat the disease but also understands how to preserve the health and how to prevent the illness in the setting of what we all live through on a daily basis: real Life, with its trials and tribulations. And so with time, I started to understand that every person's life script was somehow connected with the state of his or her health and with the workings of their organ systems. This was the beginning of understanding.

Today I am forty-five years old. Sitting in front of my Mac, I often ask myself, "What was it that really prompted me to write this book?" The answer that comes out is unexpectedly simple: "That same overwhelming desire to share my knowledge with and caring for the people who need my help." Though the knowledge and experience are now of a different kind, on a different level.

In this book I address only one health concern. It may sound simple, but as it turns out, this concern is much more difficult to treat than panic attacks or smoking cessation or chronic fatigue syndrome or insomnia. The problem we are going to tackle is this: How to live without diets and be totally happy with oneself looking in the mirror and stepping on the scale? I will let you follow in my footsteps, on my way to understanding how to treat the problem of excessive weight. In order to conquer your enemy, we will first have to identify who the enemy is and then learn our enemy's weaknesses. Only then can we try to fight this enemy. That's what my book is about. I hope that you will find it interesting. If you don't—forgive me. I am certainly not a professional writer. But I can promise you that you will find this book useful. And so, here are my experiences and knowledge of and passion for this topic, all converging in this helpful book.

CHAPTER 2

Over 97 Percent of People Who Had Lost Weight Gained It All Back over the Course of Several Years

We live in the most prosperous nation in the world. Seriously, we have the funniest commercials, cheapest foods, excess of automobiles, elevators, TVs, computers, movie theaters, gyms, clothing stores, and the highest salaries to afford it all. We eat, gain weight, and then spend a lifetime trying to lose it. What's more: we are the nation that puts up the fiercest fight against obesity in the entire world, and yet we wind up being one of the fattest.

Hundreds of diet books have been written on the subject of weight loss. Perhaps you thought this was one of them? No, this is not a *diet* book! Millions of dollars have been spent on contemporary obesity research, and most recently, the government undertook a 3.2-billion-dollar school-lunch overhaul. There is something very wrong with all the dietary advice, which an American consumer is being bombarded with on the Internet, TV, and in print media. It simply leads to more endless dieting and subsequent failure.

How did we become a fat nation? We were not born with a desire to eat fast food, to munch on popcorn while watching movies, and to snack in front of TV. Even TV itself has appeared pretty much after World War II. But with the appearance of TV in every apartment across the United States, a mass brainwashing campaign has begun. Media advertisement gets us hooked on specific foods, which are manufactured or distributed by the advertisers. The fact that obesity is now a huge problem for our country is a good indicator of how amazing is the quality of our commercial ads on TV, on the Internet, and in the movies.

And look at how we fight obesity! We are spending so much money and energy. We engage so many doctors, nutritionists, and personal trainers in this "fight." So many scientists in the labs across the country are trying to isolate the magic obesity hormone, which can be manipulated. Over fifty million Americans are members of their local health clubs. We have the highest number of gyms per capita of all the nations. What is happening here?

It has dawned on me a while ago that we are fighting the wrong guy. If TV, movies, and the Internet are so successful at getting us hooked on food, maybe it's a "sign" that we should analyze and implement those techniques, which they use to brainwash us with such ease, using our simple physiology.

How come over 97 percent of people who had lost weight on a diet have gained it all back over the course of several years?

Have you ever seen Dr. Oz pull out a sheath of cadaveric belly fat during one of his shows? This had to be an eye opener for a lot of people who have never seen tummy fat from the inside.

Unfortunately, just like smokers will not quit smoking when you show them lungs destroyed by smoke, fat people will not stop getting fat if you show them how nasty fat looks up close. Deep down, a smoker or an overweight person will whisper to himself or herself, "I am not like that. This does not have to happen to me. My great-grandfather smoked and drank and lived to be ninety years old."

To sum it up: scare tactics do not work. The only thing it does is that it contributes to our neuroses. We are already aware that we live in a polluted world, with pesticides and processed foods everywhere we turn.

So what is our diet du jour?

We are a nation of extremes and fads. There is no middle ground. We go where the wind blows. Yesterday it was Atkins diet with its bars and urine strips. Today it's the HCG diet with its injections of human chorionic gonadotrophin. Tomorrow it's a total cleanse where your colon is being stripped like a sewage pipe and then filled with different "cleansing" supplements. Or a Nutri-bullet, which is supposed to transform your food into superfood.

There is no end to brainwashing of the masses by those who want to make billions of dollars around the diet fad of the day. People struggling with their weight will put themselves through just about anything on their quest to becoming healthy and slim. At the end of the day, when all is said and done, and the dieter has gained all of his or her pounds back and then some, there is nothing but frustration, and so the vicious cycle of buying into someone's fairy-tale promises continues.

You have all seen *diet* pills advertised on TV and on the Internet. These pills work either by suppressing your appetite or by speeding up your metabolism—and sure enough, you will lose some weight while taking them. Most of these medications and supplements are very dangerous and can cause heart disease and even sudden death. FDA has banned some of them.

No matter. Billions of dollars are still being spent by brainwashed dieters on cleanses and weight-loss supplements, instead of focusing on cleansing their minds.

Some diet gurus, like your favorite hairstylists, will have you use laxative teas for weight loss. These will simply make you run to the bathroom to poop. The gut gets so lazy after using these overstimulating teas and pills, especially those containing senna or cascara, that people become constipated for the rest of their lives afterwards and cannot ever move bowels without taking major laxatives.

Money is never a deterrent for overeating either. Cigarette cost went up from 80 cents a pack in the '80s to something like $14.50 a pack today, and people are still buying them, even in these supposedly hard economic times. And to make things even worse for the obese folk, food is the cheapest, most accessible luxury we have in this country.

There are many different diets out there, waiting for you to pick them up off the shelf of a real or a virtual bookstore.

Some of these diets will call upon you to avoid carbohydrates altogether, and some will praise the benefits of intermittent fasting. Some diets will extol the caveman type of eating, yet some others will promote juices, bars, shakes, and supplements to "cleanse" you of the horrible thing that is twenty-first-century living.

In addition, the advances in Photoshop and other picture-altering software, have enabled marketing propaganda to create perfect bodies aptly positioned next to a bottle of supplements you should take, or a shake you should drink, or a powder you should sprinkle on your food, or—this is an endless list, you know.

I have divided most of the weight-loss trends and diets out there into four simplified groups. See if you can identify your past experiences with one or more of these:

(1) The first group of diets focuses on avoidance of certain major food groups, like meat, fish, breads, rice, or potatoes. As an example, Atkins diet is an intense carbohydrate restriction, which everyone is familiar with. Each of these proprietary diets has its own scapegoat of a food. Just pick a food group and restrict it because of some recently published negative press about it. Make up a name for this diet

and own it. People who put themselves through these kinds of radical limitations will often lose some weight.

However, these types of *food restrictions always lead to long-term failure*. The dieters often dream of the foods that they had to eliminate from their meals. They become nervous and irritable, by denying themselves the things they love to eat. Eventually, they "blow up like volcanoes" and regain all the lost weight. In the long run, they usually wind up with more weight than what they started off with. This creates more frustration and more defeatist attitude, which is very typical in a chronic dieter.

(2) The second trendy group of diets is based on filling your stomach with small amounts of low-calorie foods. These foods expand inside the stomach like a Chia Pet, when they are mixed with fluids. When the stomach gets filled, it sends the "I am full" signal to the brain to shut off hunger hormones from being produced.

Some of these diets will fill your stomach with the leafy greens, some will do it with juices, and yet some of the most popular European ones suggest stuffing yourself with dry oats, which will swell with water and expand. In fact, the mainstay of the currently most popular diet calls for eating three tablespoons of oat bran every day! Try it for one day: I guarantee you will be so bloated from expanded oats that you won't be able to eat anything else.

The sad result: millions of people initially losing weight and gaining it all back, with a surplus after they are done with stuffing themselves with oat bran.

(3) The third approach to weight loss proposed by the diet gurus out there is very radical. It is surgical! An entire industry has been created for this purpose. These types of procedures are covered by medical insurance only for morbidly obese, but the money has never been a deterrent for poor dieters.

One surgical approach is to cut out a large portion of your intestines, to prevent food that you eat from being absorbed. Another approach is to staple off a large portion of your stomach or to tighten it with the rubber band–like device. The idea here is to make the stomach much smaller so that eating large portions will hurt. The usual complaints after either type of surgery are pain, gas, and diarrhea. Why anybody would want to go through this agony has always been a mystery to me, but hundreds of thousands of people do it every year, having tried and failed miserably with all other weight-loss approaches.

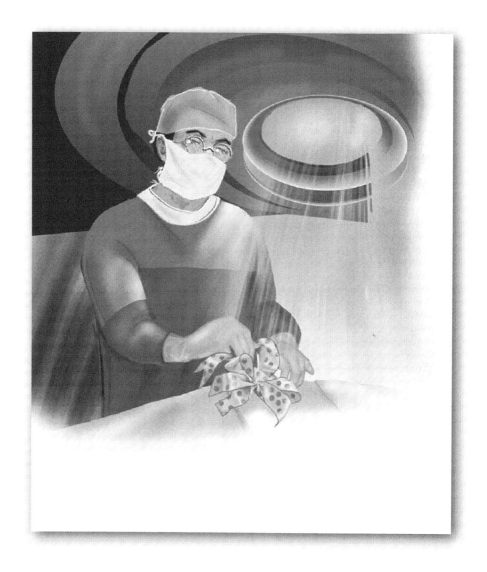

I have even heard awful stories about people gaining much more weight on purpose, to be eligible for insurance coverage for this type of surgery. Now, of all the surgical-weight-loss patients I have ever met, *no one* has emerged as a healthy and happy person. Some developed neuroses and even psychoses. Other patients developed various cheating eating behaviors, in which they would liquefy their favorite foods and thus continued to overeat.

You can surgically remove a portion of your guts, but the mind will forever be at odds with your altered body.

(4) The fourth major group of weight-loss programs emphasizes intense exercise, to burn off as many calories as possible. You will be swamped by the TV and Internet advertisements of super-lean men and women, sporting their sexy six-packs and biceps, hopping up and down to a contagious beat and demanding that you "dig deeper."

In the last few years, I have had to deal with a lot of musculoskeletal injury resulting from this type of super-intense exercise. People tear parts of their knees, including menisci and ligaments, injure their spinal discs, and wind up with low back pain and sciatica pain. They pull their necks and hamstrings.

Intense exercise hurts obese people before they see any benefit. I see these folks in my office every day. They have been jumping, squatting, and hopping for at least a month at a time, and they are as fat as they have ever been, or worse. These are real people, not commercial advertisements.

Several summers ago I went to a tennis summer camp to accompany my fourteen-year-old daughter. Very picturesque lodging in New York State's Hudson Valley. Simultaneously with a tennis camp, the hotel was also housing a large weight-loss boot camp. I would play a little tennis and then recline by the pool with a book and watch these poor obese folks, who were being exercised back and forth in the 95°F weather. They were running, jumping, squatting, and swimming in front of my face, for five to six hours every day. I also observed how they were eating, since they were sitting at the adjacent tables. They were eating like birds. It was funny and sad to watch them jiggle by back and forth day in, day out. Of course they must have lost a lot of weight over those two weeks. Unfortunately, these were the very people who would gain it all back, upon returning to their normal lives, after the boot camp. Even more disappointed with themselves and the world. Why failure?

Because the only people who can regularly function on five to six hours of intense exercise per day are professional athletes. This is their job. We have our regular nonathletic jobs and families, and a boot camp exercise routine does not fit our lifestyles.

Have you recognized the diets you have tried in these descriptions? Have you noticed how everyone you know has lost some or a lot of weight on any of the above or other types of diets and then failed to keep the weight off? Take heart—this book is meant to show you how to live a happy and fulfilling life without any *diets*.

Success is not compatible with restrictions, and truly no one wants to be a slave of dietary rules and regulations anymore. I hope that my book will stop you from being a blind follower of diets and enable you to create your own individual healthy eating decisions, which feel good *to you* and not some guy next door.

Understanding yourself is a purifying experience. It's an "Aha!" that's worth all the riches of the world. If you understand the beauty of the design you were born with, then returning to your target weight and staying there forever will feel natural and seamless.

This is what actual patients have told me:

"I turn on my TV and immediately feel like putting something in my mouth. Doesn't matter what it is, since I am not really hungry. You just go for the so-called TV snack."

"Our friends were visiting last Saturday night, and for some reason we found ourselves shopping for food the night before. Have you gone over to your friends' place, and if they didn't have a full dinner or at least some food and alcohol, you would feel like they were being cheap? We just don't want to come across as cheap."

"As soon as I sit down somewhere to watch any sport, my eyes are seeking out a bottle of beer."

What is that? A natural reflex or a throwback to ancient Roman Empire times, when people would observe the coliseum games and drink wine? Well, people were also dieting since times immemorial. Even Lord Byron, an eighteenth-century British romantic poet, has been notoriously known for his radical dietary practices, such as chewing food and then spitting it out. Imagine going to a restaurant with this guy next to you!

An anecdote comes to my mind to illustrate how such addictive food behaviors are formed. A certain doctor was treating a patient for tapeworms—large and nasty parasites—by having the patient drink a glass of milk every morning, followed by a donut. This "treatment" lasted for some time. The patient then came back to see his doctor for a follow-up, and this time he was prescribed to drink just a glass of milk in the morning, without a donut. The patient goes home and does just that. The next morning a tapeworm crawls out of the patient's behind and asks the patient: "And where the hell is my donut?"

This is a funny anecdote, but in reality, this is an exact description of a habitual ritual or any addictive habit formation, including compulsive eating.

CHAPTER 3

Journey to the Center of "Me"

We talked about the confusing world we live in, but what do we know about *ourselves*?

What Am "I"?

Is Me what I see when I look in the mirror? Or is there more?

The journey inside the human body, which I took in my anatomy and physiology classes as a medical student, opened up my eyes to the fact that, beyond our external appearance, there is a super-duper biochemical factory within.

Two different perspectives define Me.

The first point of view looks at Me as something visible and measurable and uses diagnostic tests, like blood tests and x-rays, to see how well I am doing.

The second point of view deals with things you cannot see or measure.

For the purpose of this chapter, however, let's tackle the visible and measurable Me. It is easier to comprehend, and all of us have some basic understanding of human biology from high school, which helps a lot.

The visible and measurable Me is a high-tech factory composed of "partners" called "body systems." Each partner brings a particular expertise to the table. The Musculoskeletal System/partner provides support and protection to our body and helps us to move and function the way we want. Another partner, called the Respiratory System, catches vital oxygen from the air that we breathe in and delivers it to the blood.

The partner who deals with food you eat is called Digestive System. His job is to break the food down into the small units called Nutrients. Nutrients are so tiny that they can be picked up by Blood partner and get carried to various organs. Digestive System works closely with the rest of the partners/systems, especially with the chief managing partner—the Nervous System.

The Nervous System is the boss of everyone. For example, if you are upset, you feel it in your gut almost immediately. Irritable bowel syndrome is an example of a disease, which can happen when the Nervous System treats Digestive System badly. When you are anxious, you will start breathing fast, your heart starts beating faster, and your blood pressure goes up. This is another example of how the Nervous System presides over your Respiratory and Circulatory partner/systems.

But don't get bored. I am not writing a medical textbook here. The important thing to understand is that all of our ten body systems/partners are working together from the moment of our birth until the last breath we make. Their cooperation and networking are phenomenal—there is no equivalent in our society for this kind of organizational perfection. So, all ten of our body systems are working *in unison*, with the Nervous System presiding over the body factory and executing or vetoing what it, as a boss, feels is important.

The Nervous System basically makes it or breaks it for you. A great example of this concept comes to us from ancient China's first "lie detector." Upon capturing a suspect, the Chinese would question him while making him hold some rice in his mouth. If at the end of questioning, the rice was dry—or not covered with saliva—the suspect was considered a criminal and was punished. Anxiety produced by lying would slow down the flow of his saliva, and that is why rice in his mouth remained dry.

How does the Nervous System affect everything we are? How does it get to be the almighty boss and interfere with all the other partners' work? Part of the answer came to me when I was dissecting cadavers in my first year of the medical school. I was examining the cable-like nerves, running along the arms and legs and extending to all organs of the body.

These "highways" of nerves make us look like robots, and perhaps we may even be someone's sophisticated biological machines. Large nerves become smaller nerves, and smaller nerves become tiny nerves. The tiniest ones, which can only be seen with a microscope, complete the picture of a super-complex *neural net* covering all of our body. This is how I came to see what was visible and realized the power of the Nervous System.

All business owners know that if they get sick and miss work, it is only a matter of time until their business falls apart. By the same token, when the Nervous System—the boss—gets sick, everyone in the body factory starts slacking off, and eventually things just break down. What follows is called "disease." As things get out of whack, people can get infections, develop autoimmune diseases, and feel achy and tired all the time. We don't want anything like this to happen!

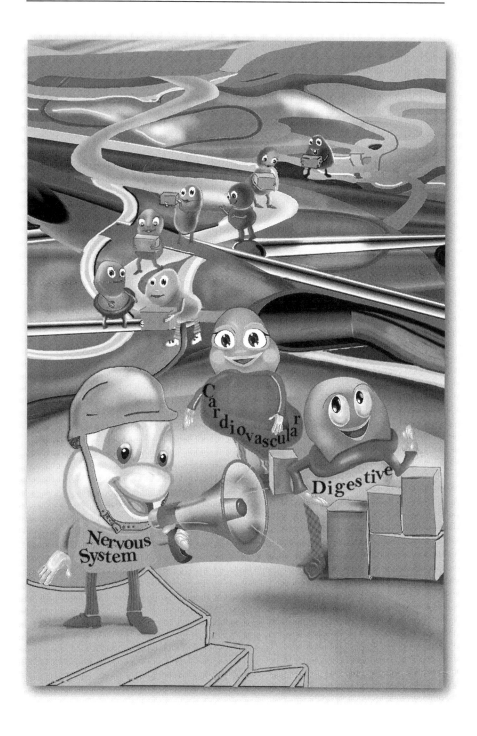

It becomes clear then that one of our main responsibilities as body owners is to maintain a healthy Nervous System. Much of this book is devoted to how to do that and how all of this is related to reaching our weight goals.

When there is a shortage of fuel and building blocks, the factory can also wind up in trouble. No factory can work without raw material, right? That's where your responsibility as an owner of these factories comes in again. A good owner must provide the state-of-the-art equipment and materials for the body factory to function seamlessly.

So you must provide healthy, optimally balanced food to your factory, to prevent breakdowns from happening. Of course, there may be situations where you need to replace a part or two, as in a cardiac-valve replacement or a hip replacement, but in this book, we will stay focused on understanding how to maintain an optimal weight and a good life, without having to put up a fight for it.

Now that we have seen that Me is a huge body factory, with ten systems/partners working in unison for our own good, let's take a closer look at this superfactory and what it does to your food.

CHAPTER 4

What Happens When I Eat?

I f you would like to understand just what happens to food after you eat it, step into your Digestive System's "kitchen."

You pick up a forkful of chicken cacciatore and place it in your mouth. You start chewing it and grinding it until it turns into a pulp. Your saliva helps you to break up this foodstuff into even smaller pieces, because that's the only way to get it absorbed into the blood at some point down the line.

It makes sense then that we should chew our food very thoroughly, in order to enable this proper digestive mechanism to take place. In fact, ancient yogis proposed that food should be chewed at least thirty-two times in tranquility and silence, without distractions. I doubt yogis were in a rush to get to work like we are, so I don't expect this kind of chewing dedication from you, folks. But seriously, chew your food well, please. It's just common sense.

The food pulp passes from the mouth into the food pipe, called *esophagus*. The esophagus is very sensitive to temperature extremes. It makes sense then that food should never be ice cold, to avoid spasms in the esophagus, which could feel like chest discomfort. Even ancient Ayurvedic texts frown upon ice-cold food or drink—they say it impairs digestion and produces mucus and congestion. Yum! Knowing this makes me sad when I see people ahead of me in line at the supermarket, starting their morning with a large iced coffee.

Anyhow, the journey of the food pulp continues down to the stomach, where it gets churned and tossed around. Many little "workers" jump in to do their part here. The most important ones are called *acid* and *enzymes*. Their job is to break the pulp into even smaller particles so that the food can be absorbed into the blood.

You are probably asking this: But what about all the acid-blocking drugs that millions of Americans take? Aren't they interfering with their normal digestive process? The answer is yes, of course they are. Just go ahead and look up the long list of side effects of two major classes of acid-suppressing medications.

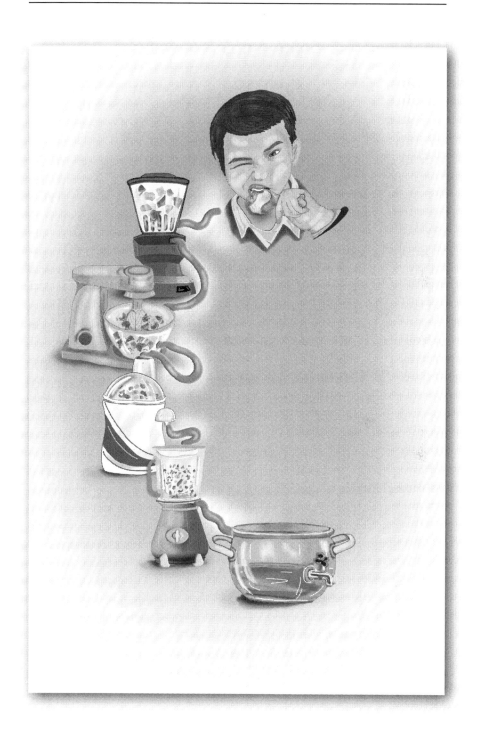

But I digressed. Back to our food-traveling journey.

Once your chicken cacciatore has been churned and cleaved into much smaller particles in the stomach, the mushy food pulp moves out into a long, folded sausage-looking pipe, called *small intestine*. Here, a bunch of little "workers" called *enzymes* jump in and start chopping this food pulp into even smaller pieces. There is even an ambassador "worker" who gets dispatched to gallbladder and pancreas to let them know that food is coming.

The gallbladder, an eggplant-looking bag, and the pancreas, which resembles a glob of cellulite, both welcome the food by releasing their own bunch of "workers," who do what? Yes, you guessed it—they just keep on breaking down this food pulp into the tiniest particles possible.

After this monumental demolition-like work is done, the food particles are now ready to be absorbed into the blood stream. Blood is like a river, which picks up those microscopic food particles from the small intestine (sausage-like factory) and delivers them to all ten organ systems:

- to the liver Cells,
- to the heart Cells,
- to the brain Cells, and so on.

So this is how your chicken cacciatore winds up arriving at your Cells. Now, let's see why our Cells need quality food to come in, not some junk.

We have an unexpected visitor—your Cell, who is wondering, "What's on the menu?"

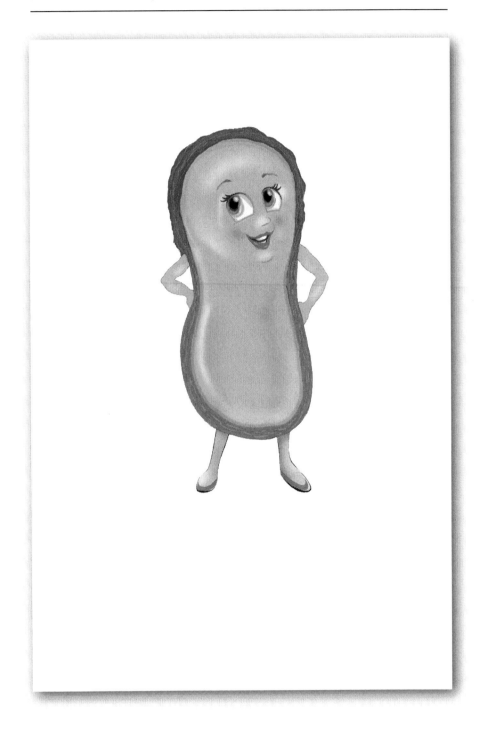

CHAPTER 5
What's on the Menu?

Hi there! Let's get to know each other: I am your Cell. There are about thirty-seven trillion of us inside you. We are like the bricks that make up your house—your body. So when you are looking at yourself in the mirror, you are staring at us—your Cells.

We are very small in size. You can only see us under a powerful microscope. But your life depends on us! All of your body systems (pulmonary, digestive, and others) are made up of us. So, this super-duper body factory of yours is really just made up of thirty-seven trillion of us, tiny little Cells working in synchrony from the moment you are born till the moment you die.

Even though I am such a VIP, my life is not easy. I work for you twenty-four seven.

And just like they substitute tired hockey players with the fresh ones, we, Cells, get regularly replaced by the new (fresh) Cells. Unlike in hockey, though, the old (retired) Cells do not come back to play.

Now, what do you need for a normal life? An apartment, a job, money, food, entertainment…

I, on the other hand, don't need all that much. For you and me to go on, I just need my food, like a car needs its gas. It may sound funny, but I take the food you feed me and make energy out of it.

That's right: I produce energy, which we—you and I—need to go on living. If you don't feed me, I will die. Whoops. Wrong. *We* will die. You and I, that is.

If you overfeed me, I have to work overtime, and I hate that, 'cause as it is, I am working like a maniac for you twenty-four seven.

When you overstuff me with food, I have to spend so much more time and effort to move the sugars, fats, and proteins around, to make sure they don't clog me up! If your doctor says that you have fatty liver, it's *me* who put the fat there. I had to move it somewhere!

If your doctor tells you that your blood sugar is high, it's *me* who has not been able to clean up the house from your excess carbohydrates. I try to clean up junk just like anyone else. But unlike you, I don't have the luxury of flexibility. Your garbage bin is at the end of the hallway. And mine is inside you!

You can reorganize your house and buy more garbage bins, *but I am stuck with you as my house*! Forever. You are me, and I am you. Period. To be honest with you, I don't wanna do all this extra job of cleaning up your overeating mcss.

Trust me; you would be much better off resting on the beach in the Bahamas, instead of being stuck here, trying to lose weight or lower your fats or sugar or whatever.

Oh well, what can I say? I cannot feed myself—I am your slave by design, and you are the one feeding me. So, please don't complain to me about your shortness of breath, difficulty walking, lack of sleep, and so on. *You* did this to us!

Well, I've got things to do. Bye for now.

If you happen to hate biochemistry and physiology, it will be very boring to read about proteins, fats, and carbohydrates unless you are a doctor or a nutritionist! However, I had to include this stuff into the weight-loss book—I am a doctor after all.

So, to be fair to you all, I decided to move the rest of this chapter into the back of the book and titled it "Appendix 1: Boring Stuff (about Proteins, Fats, and Carbohydrates)." I even tried to lighten it up with illustrations, to make it more fun to read. Should you decide to suffer through appendix 1, you would wind up having better understanding of what it means to eat a *balanced* meal and why it is important for your cute little Cells. Now, at this point you can fast forward to appendix 1 (which I am sure you are not going to do) or move on to the next chapter (chapter 6).

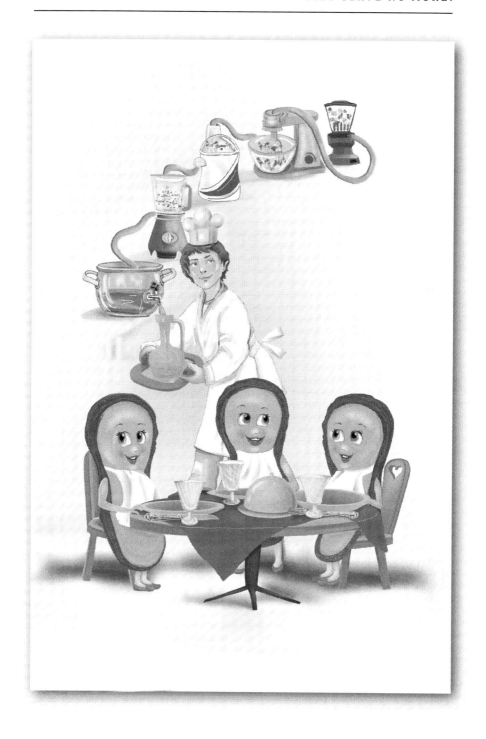

CHAPTER 6

How Do My Cells Eat?

We left off where the food you ate was broken down into carbohydrates, proteins, fats, vitamins, and minerals. The bloodstream picked up these guys from the gut and delivered them to your Cells.

The Cell needs all of this stuff to make energy. Your Cell is like a Duracell Bunny—it can work, work, and work, but only if you charge its battery with energy.

Carbohydrates, proteins, and fats line up outside the Cell as if they were applying for a job. And the Cell, being a gracious and prosperous employer, is willing to accept all three kinds of workers, but it does have a weak spot for carbohydrates.

These carbohydrates are not asking for as much "money" as fats and proteins do, but they can do the job so much better and faster! If you have a worker who costs less and performs the job more efficiently, why would you want to opt for a more expensive one? The body, with its innate wisdom, agrees and uses carbohydrates (sugars) as its preferred energy source. This is also one of the reasons why adding sugars to food makes it so desirable. Wonder why Mother Nature made those sugars so easy for the Cell to use? Perhaps because they are so available every-where around us—the fruits and the vegetables. You don't have to chase them like a mammoth for lunch and risk your life!

Let's follow carbohydrates, fats, and proteins in their footsteps as they enter the Cell. Together with vitamins and minerals, they are invited into fancy rooms, called mito-chondria, where this whole energy production business takes place. Once inside mitochondria, all these characters are told to take off their coats in a merry-go-round kind of wardrobe, while being assisted by some vitamin families, most prominently by vitamin B family.

Grateful for such warm welcome, our carbs, proteins, and fats start to show off their talents by producing a small amount of energy. This really impresses the vitamins, and they usher our workers toward their main working places—at the wall. Yes, they do have the most beautiful big wall in mitochondria!

At the wall, our workers start producing ATP molecules, which charge the Cell and fill it with energy. Now our Cell really feels like a Duracell Bunny—it has the energy to accomplish anything!

In the process, though, mitochondrial wall very quickly gets damaged with kinks and breaks. This allows for some toxic characters called "free radicals" to escape into the Cell and start interfering with everyone's seamless work. Imagine these free radicals as pirates who want to enslave your DNA by mutating it—to make it do the dirty work for them.

If your food is naturally grown, balanced with healthy carbs, healthy fats, and proteins, and rich in nutrients, like vitamins, antioxidants, and trace minerals, you are at a huge advantage. Your Cells and mitochondria will be well protected by these workers who will outnumber the free-radical pirates. Not only can the good workers stop the criminals from doing their dirty deeds but they can also help to undo the damage that has already been done.

On the basis of everything said so far, you can see for yourself that your Cells can exist and work for you only if you feed them the right way. So, it would be wise to eat healthy nutritious food, chock-full of fruits, vegetables, lean meats, and fish. If you are like me and love eating this kind of stuff, you are all set. However, if you are not a big fan, at the very least, check out appendix 2 on some recommendations for picking good sugars, fats, and proteins over bad ones, to minimize the damage to your Cells. It is better to keep your Cells satisfied—they will keep you healthy in return.

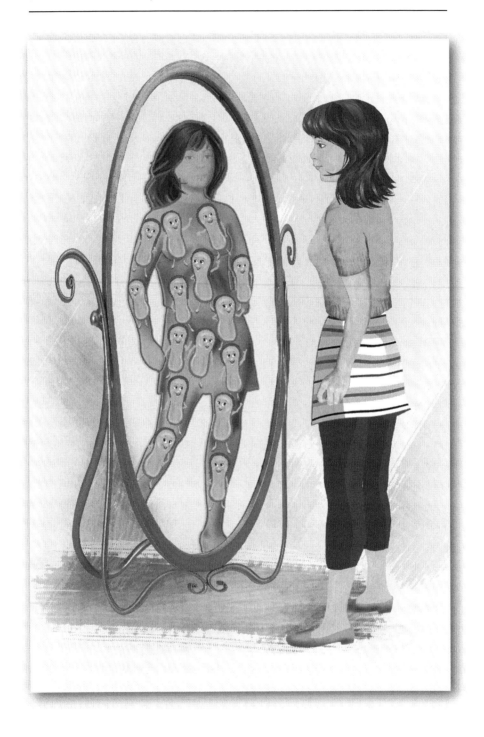

CHAPTER 7

My Cells Are Perfect—I Am Not

The world we live in treats our Cells as if there was something wrong with them. The way many popular weight-loss pills work is by stopping Cells from absorbing fat. Other dietary medications work by making you feel full after eating, by releasing certain hormones. Yet another kind of diet drugs work by blocking your appetite altogether.

No one seems to care about understanding your Cells' inborn perfection. You are being duped into buying all the food that's bad for you, because when you are obese, you become a perfect consumer of dietary pills and other medications. In fact, you are not even aware of the long list of side effects conveniently tucked into the small inserts that get thrown away with the pills' packages.

There is a reason why I took you on a journey from food to Cells, which lasted for the whole three chapters: I wanted to show you how perfect your Cells are! Your Cells have gotten you through thousands of years on this earth, by just being themselves—super-intelligent mechanisms for energy extraction from good food and fully capable of carrying out life for us humans. Did you know that 98 percent of the atoms that make up our Cells are replaced yearly? Who needs all these detoxes, which are being marketed to us in every supermarket and on every TV channel? Next time someone wants to sell you a detox regimen, tell them that the best detox is to leave your Cells alone by not feeding them junk.

In fact, the only imperfection our Cells have is *us*—their shabby owners. It is us who feed our Cells wrong things, teach them wrong things, prevent them from working properly, and interfere with their infinite intelligence. So, we are our own enemies, for not recognizing the supreme perfection of our Cells.

It is a beautiful clear summer night. And you happen to be gazing up at the starry sky. Can you sense the feelings stirring up inside you? Can you feel the longing your Cells are communicating? It is no accident you are feeling all of this: you and your Cells are made of stardust—from the same carbon, nitrogen, hydrogen, and other periodic-table elements, coupled with some mysterious energy.

By coming to understand that your Cells are highly intelligent by design, you are not committing to any religion or a cult. You are simply coming to terms with why you were born perfect and why you are such a mess today. And what's more: you are learning to tap into your birthright—your cellular integrity, to recreate your perfection.

CHAPTER 8

The Original Perfection

My grandmother once said to me, "Svetlana, you have to go back in order to move forward." I have always agreed with that wisdom. It's always better to rewind life in our memory to try to understand what milestones have brought us to where we are at today. Think back to your own kids, your nieces or nephews if you don't have any kids, or even your own childhood, if you have an amazing memory and can remember that far back.

When they are born, babies (many of us will argue that puppies too) are a bundle of sheer joy. Newborn babies exemplify what the Kaballah, the ancient mystical Jewish philosophy, calls "the beings of light." But even if you are an atheist and resent spiritual things, acknowledge this: when you walk into the elevator and you see a newborn child, it's like a curtain rises off your face; you smile at the child and feel—love.

No matter how upset you are, how tired you are, when you are standing close to your own or even someone else's bundle of joy, you feel closer to the source of this ultimate positive energy. Studies of quantum physics, which are beyond the scope of this book, help to understand how the energy of the child is affecting everyone around him or her and vice versa.

You will notice that my next illustration is not a cartoon, like all the previous pictures in this book. It is a photograph of a cute healthy baby. I inserted it here on purpose, to challenge you, dear reader, to check into your emotions at this moment. Can you sense that loving feeling taking over you? This is how the pure light of the baby transcends photo lenses, paper, and the printing process and winds up in your heart.

One day, scientists will figure out what this mysterious energy is and will give it a name.

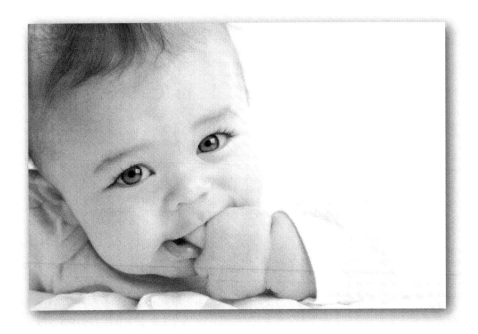

It is amazing how this precious energy fades away as we grow up and become cluttered with junk, both physical and emotional.

It's almost like pure juice, which gets diluted more and more until it becomes flavored water and not the original juice that it used to be.

Let us examine an uncomplicated life of a newborn baby. His or her life functions are simple: eat, poop, pee, sleep. Sounds familiar? One day I was overcome with the epiphany of this simplified triangle of survival functions at birth. Look at the picture of the triangle which follows, please.

It is a triangle, which all of my weight-loss patients get to know very well. These basic survival functions are wired into our old, prehistoric brain and happen automatically:

- Eating feeds our Cells.
- Sleeping allows us to pause and heal our Cells.
- Peeing and pooping eliminate the wastes that our Cells produce

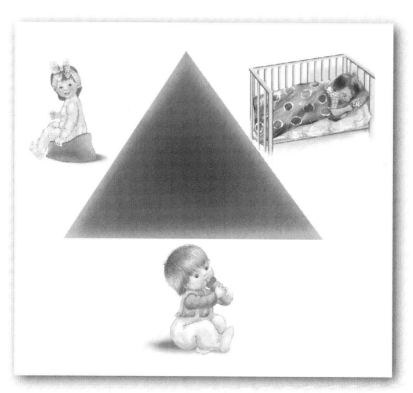

This completes a very simple geometric definition of life functions, folks. Take a look at the simple outline of the human brain as illustrated here:

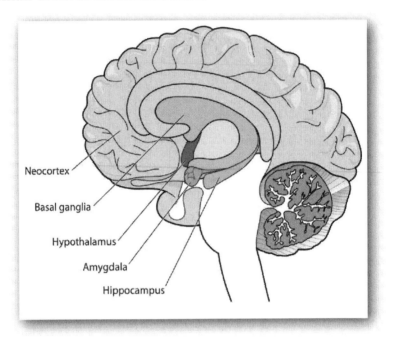

The oldest/prehistoric part of the brain is colored white. We share it with most of the animals. This part of our brain is located at the base of the skull and at the top of the neck, and that's the part of the brain responsible for the triangle of life-survival functions.

Now, back to that beautiful newborn baby. She eats every 3 to 3½ hours. Your baby is like a clock. On a very basic level, she is programmed to consume her fuel every 3 to

3½ hours, and if you don't give her a breast or a bottle, she will start looking very miserable and cry incessantly until you feed her. If you measure the amount of breast milk or formula the newborn baby consumes (and this can be easily done if you serve your milk or formula to the infant in a bottle), you will remember starting out with 2 oz., then graduating to 3 oz. After sometime you would graduate to the 5 oz. bottle, then 8 oz., then 16 oz. and so on.

"Please stop this nonsense!" an experienced parent will chide me: "There is no such thing as a 16 oz. baby bottle!"

Thank you very much for this remark, dear parent! You are absolutely right. Even the biggest babies were fed with the 8 oz. bottles.

During the first month of her life, the infant would start sucking on the milk/formula very actively and would stop and fall asleep after about 4 oz. were consumed. As time went on, your baby would fall asleep after the 5 oz., and even the biggest infant would usually stop and fall asleep after 7 oz.

But here comes an interesting observation: *a vast majority of infants would stop and fall asleep before 8 oz. were consumed.* At this point, an enthusiastic mom or dad would pet the cherubic cheek of their precious baby, trying to awaken her enough, so that she would eat some more to finish the 8 oz. bottle. I even know some parents who, out of the best intentions, would feed the milk or formula to their baby in her sleep.

The baby's brain is very well organized naturally. She gave us plenty of signals indicating that she was full and did not need any more milk or formula. These signals were as follows: falling asleep, grimacing uncomfortably, thrusting her head from side to side, or sometimes even crying. But the parents followed their own prerogative of "making sure this child is well fed" and did not pay attention to the subtle cues she was giving them, indicating that she did not need any more fuel.

It's hard to say exactly why parents tend to overfeed their babies. Those of us who were born and raised before computers invaded people's lives, and especially those who grew up in a hardship, have a notion that a baby should have a "good weight" in order to have a "reserve" to burn energy from, in case she gets sick.

So, it is only natural then that older people or immigrants will want to build that "reserve" into their babies, because you just never know what tomorrow may bring.

Or is it a plump-faced child staring at you from a Farina box on a supermarket shelf that makes you feel like your own child is underfed?

Yet other parents maybe have a well-intentioned relative or a neighbor who is quick to point out that your baby is in only 50th percentile on the weight curve. This standardization also prompts a lot of unnecessary fears in many parents who look to these weight charts for reassurance of whether their child is growing well.

Other parents simply want their babies to live up to the "perfect" pudgy-cheeked baby image on the Gerber food containers. Whatever the rationale is, most babies in the civilized societies of this world, where food is cheap and widely available, wind up being overfed.

Now, remember when you started introducing solids to your baby. In the beginning it was all blended food, in tiny jars. If you were buying prepared food in glass jars, you will recall that the sizes started at about 2 oz. and graduated to about 5 oz. for toddlers. No one has told you just how much to give, but the child would typically stop after consuming about 7–8 oz. of baby food. The same holds true for those parents who cooked their baby's first meals. Everything was blended and packaged into cute tiny containers.

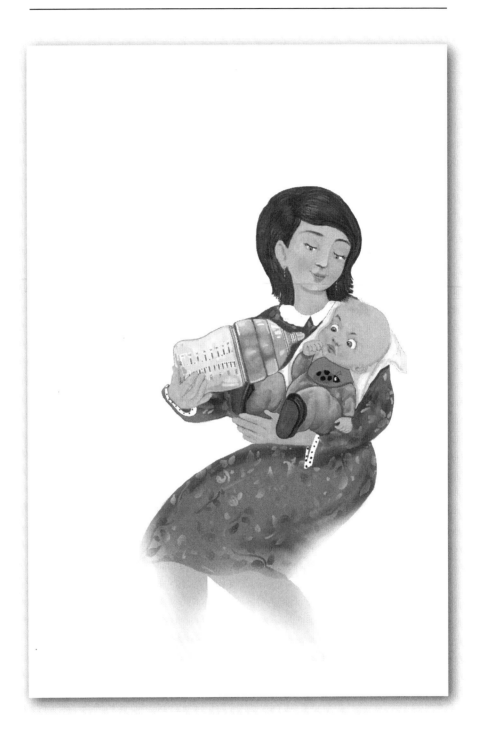

There was no parental confusion as of yet as far as the amounts we thought were appropriate for the babies at that time in their development. The real confusion started when the baby joined the adult table, whether it was in her feeding chair or in a booster seat over the regular chair. The discussion of what happens next is useless without a basic primer on how we process the world around us.

CHAPTER 9

How Do We Process What Happens to Us?

I know you must be like "Oh, I've seen this picture already!" You are absolutely right—we were using it to talk about the older part of the brain. In order to understand how we process the world around us, we need to go back to this picture. Only now we are looking at the "modern" part of the brain—the largest part, looking like a shower cap in the picture here, labeled "Neocortex."

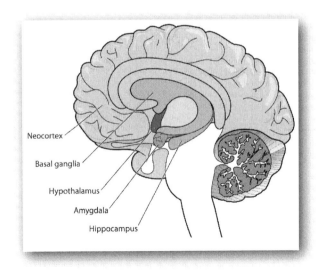

Neocortex

Basal ganglia

Hypothalamus

Amygdala

Hippocampus

Modern brain, also known as Neocortex, is like a super-computer, which processes information using all five senses, to be sure that the data get encrypted from different perspectives.

Let's recall what our five senses are. We are born with them, and they are like the antennas that translate outside information into something material, which our brain can then process and analyze. Let's review these senses:

1. Vision—allows us to see things.
2. Hearing—allows us to hear things.
3. Olfactory—allows us to smell things.
4. Touch—allows us to touch and feel things with our physical body.
5. Taste—allows us to taste things.

Everything you have ever seen and done since you were born was received by your five senses and processed by your brain. It was then deposited in your subconscious memory as a "known."

You know that the fire is hot. You know that the chocolate is sweet. You know that a game means fun.

On what day of life do the five senses start to work? An infant is almost blind at birth and can only see as far as a breast nipple or a feeding bottle. However, by six months of age, vision starts developing. Babies have to learn where things are and what they have to do to grab a bottle of milk or a pacifier, for example. It can be a frustrating process until they get it right. Visual ability evolves to an almost adult acuity at the age of three.

By contrast, baby's hearing is almost fully developed at birth and reaches a full potential by the end of the first month. That's why cooing and other tender words are so important to let the newborns know just how much their caretakers love them.

Technically, babies can hear inside the belly before they are born, and many are born with a certain preference for one type of music over the other. My six-month-old daughter would often sit on her grandmother's lap while grandma played all kinds of music. Most of the time, Rachel would try to throw grandma's hands off the keyboard, no matter what she played. Whenever she heard Mozart, though, she would freeze and just sit there quietly, listening, and not trying to push grandma's hands off the keyboard.

A baby's taste buds and food preferences start developing even before it is born, on the basis of what type of diet was being eaten by the pregnant mommy. So if mom was eating something garlicky, spicy, or salty, the child may be more readily accepting these flavors as he or she grows up.

All five of the baby's senses are very eager to participate in forming the "knowns"! Sometimes observing how this happens is endearing. For example, how many babies have you seen who play with their poop?

All of them did at one time or another. That is, until you caught them doing it. Babies' senses—visual, smell/taste, and tactile—did not object getting to know their poop. Babies could have played with their poop and sometimes even tried to taste it. Yikes!

Regardless, a "known" construct was formed in a baby's brain: poop is OK.

But then came along a screaming mom: "You cannot do that!" Mom's face is red and upset; she is raising her voice. What she is saying is hardly important to the child. What is important is the tone of the mother's voice and the upset image perceived by the baby. Now, baby's brain forms a second "known": Poop is OK but not OK to be played with or eaten.

The way our brain operates is that if a memory being built is accompanied by a strong emotion, it will be remembered stronger. In medical lingo this means more synaptic connections made between neurons. In the above example, the upset mother (angry face and raised voice) has created a more emotional, stronger memory (poop is not for eating).

On a happier note, let's take an example of how efficiently our five senses operate in a healthy child.

Meet James, a fictional kid who is four years old. He grew up in a household with a nutritionist mom and a surgeon dad. His parents have never exposed him to processed and fast foods. They were into fruits and vegetables, lean meats and fish, and have exposed their child to this diet since the very first day he started eating solid foods. The child has also been homeschooled up until now.

Now, his neighbor Ben next door is having his fourth birthday party. James's parents are fairly anxious about exposing their perfect child to other "nutritionally flawed kids," but have no choice as they live in the community and don't want to be considered weird. They drop off James at the party, and he winds up at the table with the rest of the same-age crowd.

Pizza is being brought out, and James's five senses are receiving the following signals:

1. His auditory perception (hearing) registers happy voices.
2. His visual senses (eyes) register seeing other kids' eyes full of joy and delight.
3. His olfactory sense (sense of smell) is intrigued by a new and interesting food aroma.
4. His sense of taste is tied into that smell, and the taste and image of a pizza gets assigned a precise symbolic description by the brain.
5. Finally, his hands are pulling the cheesy strands apart, following example of other kids who seem to be really enjoying themselves, playing with their pizza.

Upon receiving all of this information from five senses, James's little but very efficient brain forms what psychologists call a *gestalt*, a comprehensive symbol for pizza, which becomes forever saved in his memories accompanied by associated characteristics (yummy, warm, fun, and gooey). For consistency's sake, in this book I will call this pizza gestalt a new "known." The image of pizza will now trigger a cascade of certain emotions for James, which will undoubtedly drive him to desire pizza when he is exposed to it next time.

By the way, gestalt of the same object can change depending on the situation, and the changed perception will make a person feel differently. For example, imagine an adult dinner party. Everyone is raving about Chef X's new pizza recipe. People are putting away slice after slice, and loud munching is heard all around the house, until Chef X proudly announces that the main topping ingredient in his revolutionary recipe is nothing other than goat's balls or cockroaches or something to that effect. Everyone's gestalt is suddenly shifted. The Nervous System triggers a need to vomit, and people line up for the bathroom to do just that.

You have just formed a gestalt of how we process what happens to us.

CHAPTER 10

Hypnotized Children

How come the kids are so suggestible to what the media is "feeding" them on TV and computer and all the stuff that they are exposed to in the supermarkets, movie theaters, and parties?

Let's see. If you tell a young child, "Say something," he or she will answer, "Something." Children are literal and absorb your statements at face value. They are also very open to the "good" and "bad" qualifiers. You already know that everything that children are exposed to gets written into their permanent memory and becomes a "known."

This suggestibility peaks at around five years of age and lasts until about ten years of age, at which point it starts decreasing rapidly and levels off in the early twenties. Many evil indoctrinators around the world take advantage of the children's suggestibility by teaching them false and hate-provoking things in schools.

The ultimate illustration of how propaganda affects children's minds comes to us from Soviet history. Take a look at the boy in the picture. His name was Pavlik Morozov. The year was 1932.

Like other children of his generation, Pavlik was exposed to Stalinist propaganda, which called for identifying enemies of the state at any cost. The boy was so brainwashed that he had no problem turning in his own father for not supporting Stalin's dictatorial regime! Naturally, the Soviet government promptly executed Pavlik's father.

Look into this boy's eyes. They reveal no remorse and no pain. This is a boy who is convinced that he is doing the right thing. Such is the power of propaganda over the child's mind.

By the time children reach junior high, they are fully wired to love some people and hate others, to consider some people as heroes and to regard other people as losers. At this point, it is way too late to be putting broccoli and spinach in front of a high-school student for the first time and have them choose these or other veggies over cheeseburger with french fries.

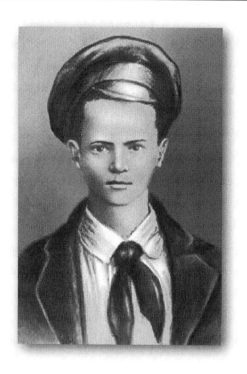

To understand why children are so influenced by brain-washing, let's look at how the child's brain operates on a wave level and compare it to an adult brain–wave activity. The next picture is a review of the major brain-wave readings as measured by an electromagnetic device called EEG.

Look at the Delta pattern, characterizing deep sleep. These waves are slow and wide. This is what brain waves of infants and children under two years of age look like when they are awake!

Now, when we adults are drowsy or daydreaming, the waves are a little faster but still quite slow, and are called Theta. The state of hypnosis is also characterized by mostly Theta and sometimes Delta states of brain waves.

When it comes to kids, children who are two to six years of age, live primarily in the Theta state, when awake.

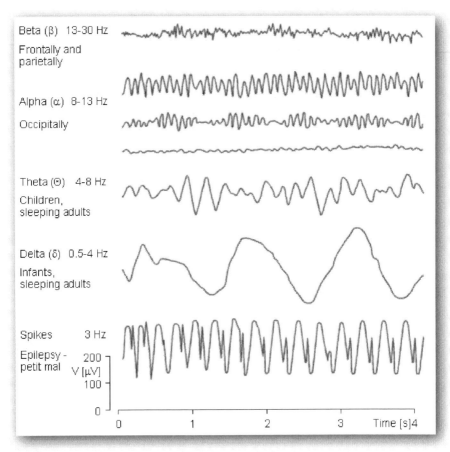

This means that our kids are literally living in hypnosis from birth until age six!

No wonder they are an open book and take everything at face value! This makes marketing job of large food industries easier than a snap of the fingers. Is there any way to escape the brainwashing? No. Children are exposed to food-related hypnosis everywhere: supermarkets, TV, movies, and the Internet.

The last fifty years have seen human life change dramatically because of advancing information technology. Unfortunately, our brains did not keep up with this evolution. Our children's brains are still wide open to an attack from anyone who decides to brainwash them, and not just regarding food.

Consider the following facts—from 577 food ads in 2011 for the most popular TV channels:

- Seventy-three percent were addressed to kids, using popular cartoon characters.
- Eighty-eight percent advertised cereals abundant with sugar content.
- Seventy-eight percent advertised fast foods.

This assault on our children's brains continues into the young adulthood. Eighty-five percent of children under eighteen are still extremely susceptible to hypnosis. Have you noticed how lately when you seat your child in front of TV he or she will likely ask you for food even though he or she had just eaten?

Parents, if you are feeding a child who is watching TV, you are feeding a hypnotized child. He is not aware of any qualities of the food you are serving him.

But don't despair. There is a light at the end of the tunnel. And it's not New Jersey. Even though we cannot undo the hypnosis of the past, we can still figure out how to achieve our optimal weight naturally and permanently.

CHAPTER 11

Bread and Circuses

I n AD 100 satirical Roman poet Juvenal wrote that the powerful of this world can win political influence over the poor people just by giving them food and entertainment ("bread and circuses," if translated directly from Latin). For centuries, the Roman government kept the populace happy by giving out free food and staging huge spectacles, like gladiator fights, to distract people from real issues. Nothing has changed over the course of two thousand years. Distraction with entertainment is a part of everything we do.

What happens to toddlers as they graduate from the feeding chair to their rightful place at the family table? Do you know someone who tends to overfeed his or her children at the family table? I surely do. As the adults are busy socializing and eating at their own pace, children are usually quickly done with their food and want to get off their chairs to go playing a game or something like that. More frequently than not, children are pressured to stay and "spend the time with the family," or they are simply stuck in their feeding chairs staring at the chewing bunch.

Did you leave stuff on your plate? I know I did. Did your parents try to make you finish the meal by saying, "This last one is for your sister, and this one is for your doggy?"

Or did they say, "Do you want to grow up strong? Do you want to be a fireman or a policeman? Then you should finish your meal"? I overheard a babysitter tell this to my son. In fact, I often overheard my babysitter reading to my older child, just to get her distracted by the story, to sneak in those extra pieces of chicken into her mouth.

But the worst thing a parent can do, in my humble opinion, is to put a computer or a video game in front of their eating child. While vacationing in the Bahamas with our two kids last year, we realized with horror that most families had their little ones staring at the cartoons and video games at the tables in restaurants.

And why should spending quality time with the family necessarily mean eating and drinking? Well, this is our life nowadays.

The moment we sit down to watch TV or listen to a band playing, even if we are standing up, we are immediately offered food or alcohol (if you are over twenty-one of course). Eating food accompanies absolutely any entertainment venue in our young or adult world. This is why any food-related business is the most thriving one in any economy. Just go outside of your home and look around at what businesses are the busiest:

- Food stores
- Cafes, restaurants, and food stands
- Movie theaters with concession stands
- Movie theaters with sit-down dinners
- Sport and wine bars with food and drink
- Cabaret with food and drink
- Stadiums with food and drink
- Comedy clubs with food and drink
- Book stores with food and drink
- Museums with food and drink
- Broadway shows with food and drink

And naturally this way of life rubs off on our kids.

My favorite, Maria Sharapova, a winner of multiple world tennis championships, a true celebrity to look up to for so many kids despite the recent scandal in March 2016, has at some point endorsed her Sugarpova candy (gummy candy, gum balls, and soft chews). The manufacturers of such candies are very well aware of how appealing candies are for kids, especially endorsed by the tennis superstar. Kids want to be like Maria. They want to somehow get close to her—at least by eating what she thinks is yummy. I doubt that Sharapova herself eats her Sugarpova candy outside of the advertisement shoots, given her 130 lb. of weight in a six-feet-two body.

In our "bread and circuses" world, ANY familiar situation is coupled with food, because it assures you of a feel-good time. These food-offering scenarios encompass your entire life, really. You could eat

- on a plane,
- in the train,
- in the park,
- on a bench,
- on a grass field,
- on a boat,

- while walking,
- on a cruise,
- in a movie theater,
- while watching TV,
- in a restaurant,
- in a café,
- at the computer, or
- on a sofa.

No matter how nutritionally sound and educated you are as a parent, if it was not you who exposed your kids to junk food, it had to be daycare or elementary school or high school or college.

"Well, my child was homeschooled," you may say.

"Good for you," I reply. But I hope that they still have experienced some sort of social interaction with other kids their age, like at the birthday parties and the local playgrounds. They had to be exposed to processed foods there, like little James we had met earlier in this book. We do not live in a vacuum. But we have the power to start communicating very early with our children and sharing our understanding of what is good for our body with them, especially since children are so suggestible when they are young.

As the primary caretaker, you are your children's most respected figure—they really trust what you teach them. So teach them the right thing. And don't forget to make your good-food stories fun and visually interesting, because as you know now, it will be all these sensory experiences that will stay with them as they are growing up. I hope that, in the nearest future, kids as young as pre-K, when they are most suggestible, will have a special program at school that deals with healthy food. It would be no less important than Reading or Math.

Earlier in this book, I mentioned that carbs are very easy to extract energy from and, therefore, can be very addictive since the body always chooses the path of least resistance, even when it comes to energy harvesting. But it is *we* who promote this addiction by saying to our little ones, "I will buy you a chocolate if you behave well," or, "if you eat this, I will give you a candy for dessert."

By offering cookies and other sweets as rewards to our kids, we are literally morphing their brains to recognize these foods as the most desirable. Taking advantage of "bread and circuses," clever manufacturers of gummy vitamins are riding the wave of record sales. Kids literally demand gummy vitamins from their parents, as a sweet reward. The way that the supermarkets are structured nowadays, there are cookies and candy strategically positioned at your ankle height so that your two-year-old can easily grab it and look up angelically at Mommy or Daddy to say, "Can I have this?"

The health-conscious parent does not have the heart to say, "No," and to deal with the consequence of a child throwing a tantrum right in the supermarket. Isn't it what the industry is counting on?

Little James is passing by the major fast-food chain, holding his babysitter's hand. In the window, he can see a happy-looking child waving his favorite cartoon character in the one hand and a french fry in the other. A free figurine of Disney character with every kid's meal! Awesome! You eat enough burgers or chicken nuggets, and you gather quite a collection. James instantly memorizes this place, its smells, the way the food looks, and very importantly, the jovial little boy in the window with a french fry in his hand. Another new "known" is formed.

When James grows up a little bit, his brainwashing will be continued by the soda-beverage companies through the ads on TV, in the movie theaters, and in the computer videos. Have you ever seen a movie in a movie theater without a soda advertisement presented to you by the coolest-looking teens or adults in the world? Drink our soda and be cool like us!

In time, James enters his adult life, abundant with TV commercials about food. These commercials are designed to be colorful and yummy looking. They are supposed to appeal to as many of your five senses as possible, and they are guaranteed to make you salivate, especially if you have not eaten for many hours. Think of all the cheese pouring onto the shrimp skewers, and all the steaks dripping with juice, topped with a yummy sauce, presented to you every five minutes while you are trying to watch the news or cartoons.

The blitzkrieg of food industry upon James's brain continues with MSG in his food takeout, aromatic essences of all sorts that are being strategically placed in the supermarkets he shops at, triggering his salivation and hunger senses with familiar and scrumptious smells.

Give them "bread and circuses,"—what a genius idea...

CHAPTER 12

The Unbreakable Web

Interview with the Neuron
(Conducted and presented by the familiar and much-
beloved Cell)

CELL: Today we are honored to hang out with a renowned citizen of the Nervous System district—my brother Neuron. You will be impressed to know that there are hundred billion neurons making up your brain. Can you please tell us what makes you guys so special?

NEURON: Well, thank you for inviting me, Sister Cell. We neurons are so complicated that humans have openly admitted that we are the least understood of all the body systems. Yet, we are the most important ones because, as you know, we are the bosses of everyone.

We pick up on everything you see, hear, smell, taste, and touch—all of your five senses. And we code this information and pass it along, one brother to another, until this information gets to its correct destination in the body. Do you like my hairstyle, Sister Cell?

CELL: Oh, this is a gorgeous hairdo, Brother Neuron! I heard that is also very special...

NEURON: Yes, you heard it right, Sister. My hair is like tentacles, like little antennae, which receive information from my brother neurons who want to stay in touch with me. I pass this information through my gorgeous long body to other brothers who are interested in getting in on it.

CELL: Oh, I see. And is it easy to get your point across to your brothers?

NEURON: I have it all down pat. I use translators: little messenger creatures who get my information across, even if it's going far away from where I'm at in the body.

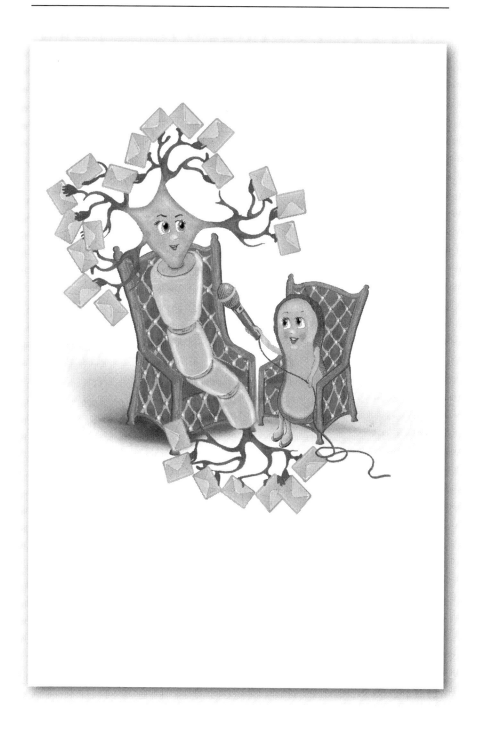

CELL: How cool is that! Is there a name for your little translator messengers?

NEURON: Yes, we call them neurotransmitters.

CELL: And is there a name for that station between brother neurons, where neurotransmitters shuttle across all this information?

NEURON: Yes, we call such place a synapse.

CELL: I heard these synapses are extremely special, Brother.

NEURON: You were always a smarty, Sister Cell. The more synapses I build between my brother neurons and I, the more efficient the flow of information becomes. Some scientist calculated that there are as many as hundred trillion synaptic connections existing in our reader's brain! Every synapse is a highway for your feelings and memories—everything you have ever known!

CELL: Hah, so everything the reader has ever learned was delivered through these synapses, all of their "knowns"?

NEURON: Yes, Sis, and the denser the net built by these synapses, just like the spider web, the stronger these habits or memories are.

CELL: Well. That's a lot for our owner—the reader—to process. Thanks very much for coming down for an interview, my darling.

Since childhood, just like little James, we associate food with very strong positive emotions and release pleasure messengers every time we eat something tasty and in a fun setting. This is how the neural webs of eating "knowns" are built so strong and durable. In fact, it is impossible to erase the old habits after they have been created. Several summers ago I came across a book called *Quantum Brain* by Jeffrey Satinover, MD, PhD. I was happy to discover that the author of the book also believed that it was impossible to unlearn something you had learned before.

We cannot undo these synaptic webs, which we have been building throughout our entire lives. Let me give you an example of "unbreakability" of synaptic connections.

You may have learned to eat with your hands as a child. You may have also learned to eat with chopsticks at an early age. Now as an adult, you may be using a fork most of the time, but it does not mean that you will ever unlearn how to eat with hands or chopsticks, right?

The important thing to understand moving forward is that the *synapses ("knowns") built in association with the strong emotional reactions will be the strongest and most memorable ones.* Remember James and his pizza? Pizza and everything else from that party he went to became wired into James's brain in association with pleasure and, therefore, will have a very strong presence in his memory. Just like you may be stopped in your tracks by the smell of apple pie with cinnamon, if your grandmother used to make it for you when you were little. By the way, many real-estate textbooks will recommend using the cinnamon-pie essence sprayed around the property that you are trying to sell, so that the buyer will instantly feel "at home."

Another illustration to the concept that emotional memories are the strongest is that fun or sad things tend to be the most memorable. We all remember what we felt on 9/11, right? And to erase this is impossible.

Do you think James will now start asking his parents to buy him pizza? I think it is very likely, if James is exposed to pizza in a similar fun-party context many times over and over again. And as if social interaction with other kids was not enough, little James happened to be in a supermarket last week with his babysitter, and here is what he saw: colorful and fun-looking boxes with cereal and all kinds of chips and crackers. Crackers looked like funky animals and fish, and the boxes of cereal had James's favorite Disney character drawn on it, in 3-D! The babysitter said, "All kids find toys of their favorite cartoon characters if they eat enough cereal to get to the bottom of the box!"

Wow! Not only is this appealing but it's also very exciting to little James. He starts coveting cereal even if he has never tasted it before. An incomplete "known" is formed, as not all five senses were used to materialize it, but imagine how strong a memory will form when this takes place. This week. Next week. At a friend's house. In a daycare center.

On a playground. Rest assured it will take place, because we don't live in a bubble.

The synaptic webs we have built in childhood and adolescence are unbreakable, but the beautiful thing is that we can just keep building the new, desirable webs as much as we like.

CHAPTER 13

Creating New Reality/New Synaptic Webs

In his ageless book *Alice in Wonderland*, Lewis Carrol beautifully illustrates that most people don't really believe that they can achieve a significant change in their lives:

> *Alice laughed. "There is no use trying," she said. "One can't believe impossible things."*
>
> *"I daresay you haven't had much practice," said the Queen.*
>
> *"When I was your age, I always did it for half-an-hour a day. Why, sometimes I've believed as many as six impossible things before breakfast."*

Mao Tse Tung once said, "In order to learn how to swim, one must swim." Mao is certainly not my favorite historical figure, but he was right about swimming. I will dilute his image with one my favorite folktales, as follows.

Two little frogs fall into a large container of cream. One of them screams, "We are going to drown!" The other says, "We'll see about that. Let's try to get out of this mess." The first frog quickly gives up and drowns, while the second frog keeps on swimming, turning, moving, and psyching himself up to stay afloat. After a while, he is exhausted and cannot move anymore. But lo and behold: there is ground under his feet. The persistent little frog turned a container of cream into butter!

So can you do it? Can *you* finally stop being a Diet Slave knowing everything you know now about the way your body and Cells work, and knowing your brain's weaknesses exploited by the world we live in? I think that, in order to answer this question, you should continue your journey into this book and see for yourself.

Of course, the main obstacles we have as human beings on our quest to learning a new eating habit is laziness, the desire for instant gratification, and the fear of failure. We turn to our conditioned "processed" thoughts as an easy way out, just like we pick up processed foods on the fly in the supermarket. But, as Dr. Satinover puts it in his book

Quantum Brain, "if the *new pattern* is repeated deliberately, diligently and frequently; and if the old pattern is willingly avoided for a long time, then the very old habits of thought, feeling, and action will slowly weaken as the newer ones grow strong" (abbreviated).

The folk wisdom agrees almost word for word: "If you don't use it, you lose it" and "Practice makes perfect."

If you were born left-handed and raised in a socialist dictatorship like the Soviet Union or China, for example, you had to undergo an evil process of learning to write with a "proper" right hand. You all remember the tears, the despair, and feeling like a stroke victim whose limb does not want to move properly. Sleepless nights, more torturous writing, more tears, and failure—more repetition and more writing with the right hand, until one day when you were writing with your right hand. Interestingly today, I still only write with my right hand, while all the other functions, including drawing, holding a knife, and putting on makeup, are still done with my (originally dominant) left hand. What about you?

Watching athletes train for an event or observing ballet dancers rehearsing for a performance helps to reaffirm the idea that if you exercise your synaptic webs over and over again, they grow to be remarkably strong. The athletes' and dancers' outstanding achievements are a result of endless rehearsing a particular movement or a stretch or a jump. If they psych themselves up in the process, it helps, and the memory of a perfected performance becomes strongly cemented in their memory.

How can one psych himself up to do something with pleasure?

Emotions are created by tiny neurotransmitter molecules. There are receptors for these molecules throughout our body, not just in the brain, and most are actually located in the gut. You all know the expression: "I feel it in my gut" or "I have a gut feeling about it." This is literally true. And for that very reason, all antidepressant medications have nasty side effects on most organs in the body, especially the gut.

This is also the reason why the very process of eating food promotes positive emotions. Since we are naturally seeking to experience good emotions, the easiest way to get them is by eating.

What got me fascinated with the molecules of emotions was the research of a former chief of brain biochemistry at the National Institute of Health, Candace Pert, PhD.

Dr. Pert discovered opiate receptors in the brain and has written many scientific articles and several wonderful books on the matter of emotions. She described how millions of different receptors are sitting on the Cells. These receptors are like unique tiny antennae, which are patiently waiting until an appropriate chemical comes along and fits into them perfectly, just like a key would fit into its unique lock. No, I think a better way to describe this unique fit is to say that the neurotransmitters and their receptors are like pieces of the puzzle that fit together perfectly.

So, a tiny chemical called a neurotransmitter (green envelopes in the neuron illustration) delivers its chemical information to the receptor, which then transmits this message deep within the Cell, triggering a chain of biochemical reactions within the Cell, of either a positive or a negative nature.

A good example of a neurotransmitter in action is an endorphin molecule. It is our body's own opium, so to speak, since it attaches to the same receptors that narcotics like morphine bind to. You have also heard of larger neurotransmitters: serotonin, adrenaline, dopamine, and others. As a matter of fact, every time we feel positive emotions (like fun and excitement), we experience a specific rise in serotonin and dopamine levels in our blood, corresponding with each shade of emotion. Experiencing emotions is the result of a very complex interplay of many neurotransmitters. A "cocktail" of molecular joy is unique and different for each emotion that comes over you.

Let's see how our five senses are involved with creating positive emotions. Imagine sitting on the porch and blissfully sipping on the best cup of coffee in the world. The emotion you feel is a result of all five senses contributing their information to the brain.

Let's say, before you even had a chance to get to your cup, your ears have registered "Honey, your coffee is on the table!" Your eyes have registered a beautiful mug with richly colored coffee in it. Your nose has sniffed the unmistakable hazelnut (why not?) aroma of this beverage. Your tongue has conveyed the unique aftertaste after swallowing the first gulp. Your hands are clasping the warm cup holding this coffee.

All of your five senses are creating inputs, the same way that the five different journalists are relaying their reports of the same event to the central news station.

It's like a movie being filmed with five cameras simultaneously and then being edited. The end results of all the edits are fused together and wind up on the same film. Once the brain edits the information it receives from all five senses, it then registers the big picture and triggers chemical reactions (little green envelopes in the neuron illustration). These chemical reactions generate different emotions you are feeling: "Mmm, what a delicious coffee! Thank you, my darling!"

This moment of bliss has been brought to you by brother neurons joining their hands in millions of synapses. There is no limit to how many of these synapses can form. The more synapses there are, the stronger the blissful memory of sipping on that coffee: "Mmm. Fantastic!"

I may be repeating myself here, but it's very important to note that whatever has already been registered by the brain cannot be erased. And the more senses involved, the stronger the information recorded.

If the auditory sense did not participate here (your honey did not let you know that your coffee was on the table), the coffee would not taste any less delicious. Perhaps you would not be smiling at the fact that you are so lucky to have your sweetheart. But the overall emotion would be—shall we say—less colorful. And your perception of this cup of coffee would be more like a good draft rather than a full-fledged painting.

In fact, a recent research in Germany found that blind-folding a group of people who were eating ice cream resulted in feedback that described ice cream as less pleasant. It's not that the blindfolded folks disliked their ice cream. No, they enjoyed it, but less intensely than their counterparts whose sense of vision was present in the experiment. This is what I meant by a less colorful experience, when not all five senses participate.

Interestingly, in another smaller study, the researchers found that those participants who ate their lunch blind-folded ate the portions that were 22 percent less than the portions of those who could see what they were eating. I hope you see the irony in the fact that deleting one of the five senses reduced the portion eaten by one-fifth in this experiment.

Just like a positive emotion, like hearing your beloved calling you with a cup of coffee, can strengthen your positive perception of an object, in this case coffee, the negative emo-tion will cause predictable results. Even if only one of the five senses is suddenly conveying an unpleasant emotion, the overall perception of an object will be affected dramatically. A cup of coffee offered by someone you resent will make this beverage tough to swallow. So, emotions are always there,

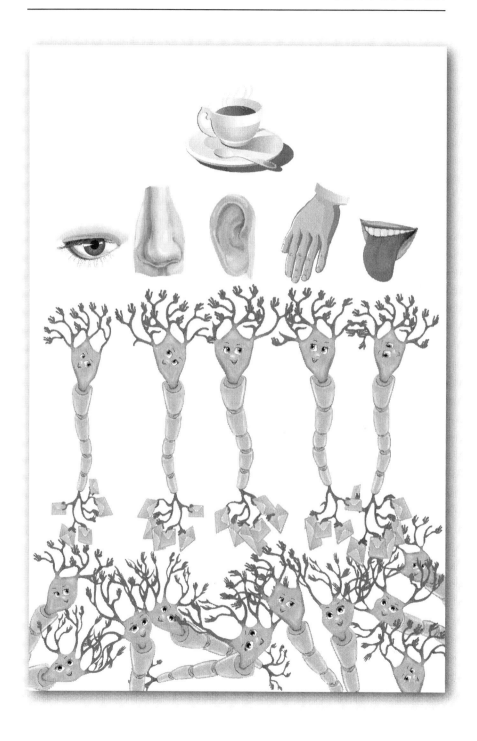

accompanying our five senses, feeding into them, and getting nourished by them.

Years ago, an old patient of mine had suffered a horrible flu, and her smelling and tasting nerves were severely damaged. The old tastes as she knew them—salty, bitter, and sweet—were gone! Tasting dry versus wet was gone, too!

In fact, when she put anything in her mouth, it had a completely foreign feel to it—her tongue felt "something," and that something was completely new and "unknown," without any point of reference. My patient could not smell anything. She could smell neither flowers nor the freshly cut grass, nor the ocean. She could not even smell the unmistakable scent of her child. But the scariest thing was that she almost died in a fire, after her kitchen towel was sent ablaze while she was cooking. Though she could not smell a thing, she happened to miraculously turn her head and notice a burning towel. Her life became a living hell.

I could never forget how she frequently came to the office crying and asking me if she had gone crazy. She told me she *remembered* the taste and the smell of the fried meat. But now it did not have *any* taste. Now, she could not even taste the difference between a pizza and a cake or between a candy and a pinch of salt. Not even between a piece of chocolate and a spoonful of soup! My patient found herself in the midst of a whole new and strange world.

Today I understand that, receiving information from just three instead of five senses (since my lady patient lost her senses of smell and taste), her brain could not match this information up with the symbols of the previously recorded life scenarios ("full paintings"), as *they* were recorded using all five senses. This *newly received information from just three senses—the so-called draft*—for someone who was used to a "full-fledged painting" *required a new "known" symbol* to be formed and recorded by the brain. And it had to be repetitively memorized.

It is only now that I understand just how vital it was for her to vent her frustration and despondence to me in the office. And no wonder they say that time heals. Time truly heals, as the new scenarios and symbols were being registered and recorded by her brain. This required repetition and years, and my patient survived only thanks to her infinite persistence and hope. Faced with her horrible physical limitations, she accepted her new reality and started living her new life and making new symbols and memories. It was then, when she stopped thrashing around in her mind's old memories, that she found her peace.

I can only imagine a person who is deaf or blind, or even both deaf and blind, living in this world and processing it through the remaining senses. Such person could easily have a disabling flu like my patient did. I think he or she would most likely go through the same torturous process my patient went through and would arrive at accepting his or her new life and making new emotions and memories. Am I sure about that? No. For the only sense left to such an unfortunate person would be the sense of touch. Could he or she create the new "knowns" and emotions generated by touch? I can only hope so. I think the sense of touch would maintain that material connection to the outside world, without which we are but a soul.

Why am I telling you these stories? No, this book is not about complications of influenza virus. It's about losing weight naturally, without diets, and keeping it off. My patient's journey had a tremendous impact on my understanding of how our brain processes the outside world. And I would like to share this knowledge with you because *your* task of learning healthy eating ways and making them your own is infinitely easier. Most of you are lucky to possess the arsenal of all five healthy senses. And you know that your brain is amazing at creating *new* symbols, emotions, and new synaptic webs. The toughest parts will be repetition and persistence. Don't worry; you can move mountains with powerful tools like five healthy senses, never mind reaching your simple goal of losing unwanted weight!

You may be looking at yourself in the mirror and thinking, "To hell with all the diets; I am so fat anyway! At least I enjoy eating whatever I want and whenever I want. Pizza, ice cream, and chocolate make me feel better!" This may be your old scenario, which has accompanied you through many failures and disappointments.

But I would rather make you realize just how powerful you are. I know that your inner resources are endless, even if you may think you are losing your battle with yourself. True, your eating habits have been affected by the world you live in. You cannot undo that. But there is no question in my mind that you are capable of creating a new reality for yourself, by building new synaptic webs. By tirelessly revisiting these webs, you can make them your own.

I will try to help you write your own new reality, in which you care deeply for those who depend on you, like your Cells, or for someone else, intimately involved with your good eating habits. We shall see.

CHAPTER 14

Introducing ID and SUPEREGO

I n 1874 Dr. Ernst Wilhelm von Brucke, an Austrian phys-
icist and a founder of the science of psychodynamics,
published his lectures on physiology, in which he postu-
lated that all living organisms are energy systems governed
by the first law of thermodynamics. This law, which we all
learned in high-school physics, states that the total amount
of energy in any given physical system is always constant and
that energy can be changed but not destroyed. What follows,
said Dr. von Brucke, is that when energy is moved from one
part of the system, it must reappear in another part.

This publication made a huge impression on a young
medical student by the name of Sigmund Freud, who was
rubbing shoulders with his "academic advisor" von Brucke
and even did some research with him at his physiology lab
at the University of Vienna.

Freud devoted his entire life to exploring the very field of psychodynamics, which von Brucke had pioneered. He figured that "if the energy inside our mind travels and changes shapes and flavors, let me create my own system, which can serve as the foundation for human behavior." Freud felt that our behavior and feelings were powerfully affected by the unconscious motives rooted in our childhood experiences and seated in the old brain.

Unfortunately, in their research, both von Brucke and Freud referred to the only kind of physics that was known to them at the time—classical mechanics. Imagine just how thrilled they would be to learn about the discoveries of the new discipline called quantum physics and how it would broaden the energetic foundation of their psychodynamic work!

So Freud, with his tendency to organize and classify things, divided the mind into conscious and subconscious domains. He called his mind players ID, EGO, and SUPEREGO.

ID represents the most instinctual, inborn tendencies. It exists exclusively on the subconscious level. ID does not care about consequences of doing something inappropriate. Its function is to multiply/procreate and enjoy yourself in the process.

If you ask your friend, who is a diabetic, why she is gulping down a chocolate Yahoo drink, she will tell you this after she awakens from the diabetic ketoacidosis coma: "I don't know what came over me." What came over her was ID with its lifelong sweet tooth.

If ID were the only thing controlling our lives, we would all become sex perverts and druggies. Clearly, some kind of censorship part of the mind is needed to keep us in check. Freud called this censoring part of our mind SUPEREGO. This part is a by-product of being brought up in a particular cultural environment and is kind of a "conscious citizen" figure.

SUPEREGO tries to make sure that the person does the right thing. It's like your mom who is always telling you what to do.

Let's say you are a guy, at a party, standing alone with a drink, on a patio in moonlight. There is a drop-dead gorgeous stranger approaching you, draped in sexy clothes, with a glass of wine in her hand. She is looking right into your eyes, and your ID revels from potential possibilities. What a dream come true! You are on fire!

All the while, your SUPEREGO is screaming bloody murder: "You can't listen to your primitive self! You are married to your high-school sweetheart and have four kids in private school. Your mother-in-law will cut your throat with a surgical scalpel she will steal from her neurosurgeon husband!"

Who do you think will win, your ID or your EGO?

Oh, to be or not to be...

Sometimes, the choice is clear, especially if ID and SUPEREGO are agreeing on something. For example, if I travel to a street market in Bangkok and see fried insects being sold on the street as snacks, I won't salivate but instead will feel rather nauseous, because my upbringing did not expose me to eating insects. By the same token, if an Indian man sees an Eastern European man eating a sausage made from cow's blood, the Indian will most likely feel sick to his stomach because his SUPEREGO considers it a savage and unholy practice, on the basis of his cultural upbringing.

EGO part of the Freudian mind system functions like an ambassador, shuttling messages between ID and SUPEREGO and registering the state of conflict or peace between the two, but it is SUPEREGO that analyzes any given situation and makes decisions, such as the following:

- To be or not to be?
- To cheat or not to cheat?
- To let my anger out or to hold it back?
- To stay in this job or to shut the door in my boss's face?

Freud felt that when a person's primitive urges were in opposition to his code of morals, like ten commandments for example, a person would feel very torn within himself. Freud called this conflicted state a "neurosis."

In the context of weight loss, if you are experiencing a constant craving for something but cannot indulge in it, after a while you emerge as a very stressed-out person. A common example is a person craving sweets but living on an Atkins diet, which is very low in carbohydrates (sugars).

This frustrated person is easily startled, irritated, and cannot fall asleep at night. His friends and family describe him as "always on the edge," and "emotionally volatile." A chronic dieter has a high cortisol level, which can lead to heart disease, diabetes, stress ulcers, and depressed immune system.

So, if you are on *any* diet, you are essentially creating a conflict between the ID, who is looking out for your feel-good status and survival, and the SUPEREGO, which recommends restrictions.

You will feel much better if you stop denying yourself the food you are craving. If you like to eat meat, you will happily notice that you have fangs. Maybe you were meant to sink your fangs into steak. Personally, I like to sink my fangs into fish. For someone else, it may be tofu. If you happen to like meat, don't try to turn into someone who is a vegan. You will start craving meat until one day you will find sinking your teeth into it harder than ever.

I knew a ballerina who was hardly eating anything at all, because her male stage partner would curse her out every time she ate as little as half an apple before dancing rehearsals. Her partner had to lift her a lot, and he felt her every added ounce of weight, even that half apple's weight. She confessed to me that her life was nothing but a stress ride, and she was dreaming of food even while having sex. Her biggest wish was to retire at thirty-five so that she could finally eat "like a normal person."

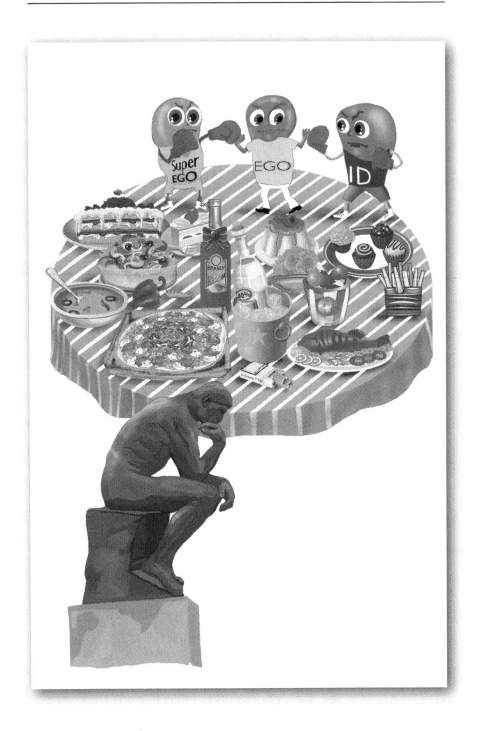

I have also known many athletes who retired from a very intense athletic activity and immediately expanded like balloons. Many gymnastics and figure-skating coaches belong to this camp of people, who were denying to themselves the pleasure of what they wanted to do for decades and then finally let themselves go.

ID was set out, by design, to experience the bliss of life and will resent any restriction or conflict. This is an important truth all dieters should realize.

People who ignore their internal conflicts are always stressed out because the world seems very unfair to them. The dark lenses through which they choose to process the world around them are making these people commit to bad decisions. For example, they will scream threats and curses in traffic at someone who is cutting in front of them. In fact, you can have the nicest person, who would normally not hurt a fly, get so worked up in a traffic jam that he or she may get into a violent altercation with the other drivers and wind up detained by the police. The world is designed to simultaneously contain the bad and the good in us. But the choice of what to become is ours.

The rest of this book will be dedicated to finding the way to eliminate the conflict and promote peace between the ID and SUPEREGO. Knowledge is power, and the more we can understand ourselves, the sooner we can achieve this balance and succeed in our goal of losing unwanted weight naturally and maintaining it forever.

CHAPTER 15

Mind Games

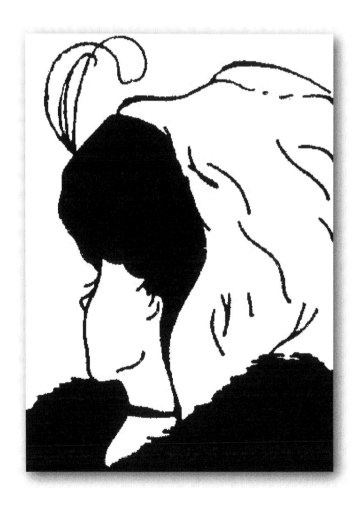

What do you see in this picture? Do you see a face of an old woman or a young woman?

You are capable of seeing both but only one at a time. By the same token, we can perceive a flower, as beautiful versus ugly, or we can perceive a color as warm or cold.

Here is another example of how we perceive things.

Is one hair a lot?

Not on your head—you have thousands of others. The idea of one hair on your head does not stir any feelings.

What about one hair in your soup?

Whoops. This image triggers disgust. Please tell those chefs to wear hair caps!

Your mind has options to interpret appearances or food choices, or anything else you come in contact with, whichever way it pleases. Possibilities for interpretation and perception are endless, but we usually choose one perception at any moment in time, thanks to our free will. Our mind creates endless scenarios for every action and reaction. Let's say you are a woman, walking down the hallway to your workstation on a Monday morning. A male colleague passes you by and remarks, "Nice hair, Jane!" There are endless ways you can process this information, and just as many ways it will make you feel:

- You could think, "He really implied that my hair is a mess," and feel insecure and hurt as a result.
- Or you could think, "This man can really appreciate just how beautiful I am," and feel flattered.
- Or you could think, "He is hitting on me!" and feel either happy or annoyed depending on how you perceive that man.

The list of possibilities you can pick for yourself is endless. These mind games always participate in how you eat and in pretty much every move you make.

Several years ago, while vacationing on Marco Island, Florida, my then three-year-old son, Marc, was eating ice cream with me, seated outside the ice-cream shop. Inside the shop a family of five was seated: parents and three kids. One of the boys had all the features of the Down syndrome. Marc pointed at this kid in the window and said, "Mommy, this one is the most beautiful one." I almost cried at how my son's pure consciousness, barely touched by brainwashing, has stated his truth, bringing out emotions so different from what most of the adult world would feel.

But as we grow up, our upbringing conditions the lenses through which we look at the world. By the same token, our capacity to see the same object from various perspectives can also make us perceive certain foods as appetizing versus disgusting. Even though it is yet unclear, neurologically speaking, why exactly some people's minds make a preference of seeing something first, an old woman or a young woman in the above picture. What is clear though is that our upbringing eventually influences the way our brain will process the information perceived.

If I introduce healthy grilled fish, meat, and vegetables to my five-year-old and associate it with a sense of goodness, comfort, and homey togetherness and make sure that the child is exposed to this type of fare more often than not, the child will grow up to associate an image like the one shown here with a definition of awesome dinner.

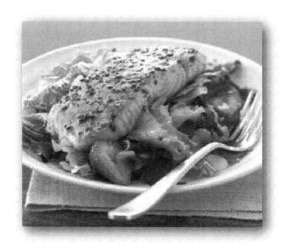

When I was growing up in Ukraine, my grandfather used to place a slice of lard on a piece of bread and eat it slowly, savoring its flavor. He survived World War II and lived through many starving times, and for him lard on the bread was the ultimate reminder that life was good. It imbued me with a certain amount of awe, to see him pick up the fallen crumbs off the table after he ate and put them in his mouth. Like any child who mirrors her family's behavior, I was delighted to share these meals with my grandfather whenever I visited him. Of course, the same kind of lard would make most of you nauseous at first sight, if you were not exposed to it as a child. But for me an image of lard on a piece of black bread will conjure positive feelings because this "known" cannot be erased.

The same holds true for the sausages made of cow's blood, which were considered a delicacy when I was growing up, even the mention of which would offend my Indian friends, who consider a cow to be a holy animal. But for me, an image of a blood sausage still brings a feeling of familiarity and acceptance, when I see it served in Russian restaurants in Brooklyn.

However, let's say I will place three familiar images in front of me when I am about to eat. The upper left image is lard on a slice of bread, the upper right is sliced kielbasa, and the lower centered is grilled fish with veggies. I apologize for the lack of color (which totally changes our perception by the way), but publishing this in color would have made this book unaffordable for most people. What would I choose?

My hand would naturally reach for grilled fish. Why? I have made neither the left nor the right choice for many years, but the images are familiar and not repulsive to me. They are my "knowns," which cannot be erased.

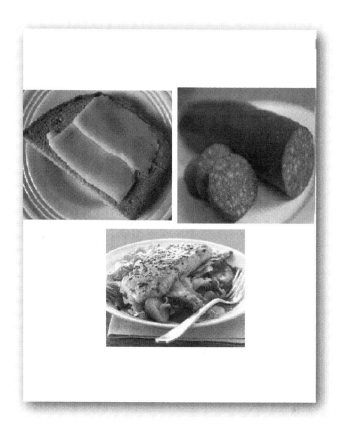

If we imagine our memory as stacks of shelves, then blood kielbasa and lard on the bread are likely neatly tucked away on the farther or harder-to-get-to shelves.

Visualizing these images does bring up Grandpa and sweet memories of childhood, but my SUPEREGO, the decision maker of my mind, is feeling quite neutral toward these remote memories and drives my hand toward the fish platter, as a comfortable compromise between itself and my ID, whose preference is simple: "I like eating."

The salmon (or it could easily be grilled chicken) is what I have been eating on a regular basis for years. And that's the new reality I have created for myself—my "known," which I am most frequently exposed to nowadays. Many brother neurons have joined their hands every time I've sat down to eat this type of platter to form their unbreakable synaptic web. For my brain, this became the highly exercised path of least resistance, and it was coupled with positive emotions of socializing or having conversations at the dinner table. Think about this.

As an aside, here is an anecdote about differences in upbringing. I once froze in front of my Indian classmate's apartment with a swastika on the door. To a Jew this meant a death threat, and to my friend this meant a sacred Hindu good-luck charm, kind of like our Jewish mezuzah.

Some of you might find it despicable that certain French people eat frogs as a delicacy, but this image would certainly provoke nothing but salivation in most Frenchmen dining in a French restaurant. In many Asian cultures, the street vendors sell popular fried insects, the very sight of which makes me cringe. But they are tasty and full of protein, many of my Asian emigrant friends may counter. I think you can pretty much tell where I am going with these examples.

Indeed, the way we perceive the world in general, and food in particular, depends on where we come from culturally. Hell, some people in New Guinea ate their diseased relatives' brains until the 1960s, when an American and an Australian doctor traveled out there and explained to the natives that it was their cannibalistic eating habits that were responsible for them dying from kuru—an incurable neurologic disease. But for the New Guinea natives their delicacy might have meant for them what black caviar and champagne means to us, Westerners. Oh, those mind games…

Babies start their cultural "initiation" very early, as soon as they are able to run around the house. Potty training is a great example. It starts earlier in some countries and later in others. The fact that a child must pee in a designated area (potty), instead of peeing in their diapers, is also geographically dependent. Some tribal people in rural Africa relieve themselves in the bushes, and in some rural and underdeveloped areas of Eastern Europe and Latin America, it is totally acceptable as well.

One of my patients who emigrated from Ukraine once told me that he saw his three-year-old daughter pee under a tree, just like a little doggie would. Horrified, my patient turned to his babysitter, who herself grew up in the Ukrainian boondocks, and she confessed to him that this was how she herself grew up. There was no point in going home if you felt like relieving yourself, she said, as long as there were trees or bushes around. So much for the early cultural initiation affecting the way we grow up to behave.

Teaching a child to take a shower at least daily is another example of how societal norms build our adult behavior. Many emigrants from the third-world countries have to learn to use a deodorant when they come to the United States because they realize that they have a body odor, which may be offensive to people around them. Back in their native countries, many immigrants have experienced a shortage of water and were not as fortunate as we are to be able to take several showers a day. A patient who was an emigrant from Moldova told me that growing up she had access to water only from midnight till 6:00 a.m. Today, my patient is living out a different reality, in which there is plenty of shower opportunity. The old synaptic web has not been erased, but the new one has been created and reinforced day in and day out.

A funny story comes to my mind, told by a long-time patient of mine. She was brought up in a religious Jewish family, with a strict taboo against pork eating. One day she was at a party where everyone's plate was prefilled with appetizers. She forgot her glasses at home and could not see very well. She had overheard several people in the room talk about pork, and even though she had no idea what they were talking about, her brain made a note of it. Her brain had subconsciously prepared for an assault by a forbidden taboo that pork represented.

When she picked up her appetizer (which in the end turned out to be grilled cheese coated with bread crumbs), she assumed it was pork from the way it looked. Unsure of herself, she poked it with a fork and tasted a tiny piece. She felt "pork" coat her mouth and analyzed the taste, but through the "pork lenses," her brain conveniently extended to her at that moment. "Pork!" she concluded with disgust and set the plate down, just to find out several minutes afterward that the appetizer was in fact her favorite grilled cheese...

So much for the mind games.

Is it possible to change any rules of these games? Let's see. You cannot change the ID as it's built into you, just like your heart or your liver are. You cannot change the EGO because its ultimate goal is to mediate between the ID and SUPEREGO. But what about your SUPEREGO—that is, the collection of symbols or "knowns" since you were born?

Granted we cannot erase them, but we can keep recording the new ones, forever, until our last breath. If newly recorded "knowns" are pleasing to ID and satisfy SUPEREGO, they get a priority (easy) access on the memory shelves, as far as recall is concerned, and the balance is achieved. The more we experience these feel-good "knowns," the harder it is to live without them. So, it looks like things can be worked out with SUPEREGO!

Think about how hard it would be to lose a loved one, especially if they lived with you or close to you, in the same city where you have been spending time together on a regular basis. Such loss would feel more painful than the loss of a loved one who lived in a different country, because in the latter case the "knowns" of taking rare walks together or looking into each other's eyes would be pulled from the dustier, more remote memory shelves.

Somewhat less dramatic example would be your teenage child going away to a college in a different state across the country, or even abroad. What an awful time, people say. It probably takes months to get used to not being able to put your child to bed, not to be able to hug them and ask them about their day at school.

One elderly patient who emigrated from the former Soviet Union in the '70s told me about her daughter whom she had to leave behind. As it happened, it took fourteen years for these two to reunite. When my patient left the Soviet Union, her daughter was only twenty-one, and all these years they were communicating only through letters. When her daughter was finally granted permission to leave the Soviet Union to come to the United States, she was thirty-five years old. My patient was ecstatic, but after another ten years went by, she confessed a "horrible secret" to me during one of her visits to the office. You see, she loved her now forty-five-year-old daughter who was reunited with her after that horrible separation. However, my patient would some-times feel wistful, recalling the images of the twenty-one-year-old girl, whom she had left behind at the train station in Russia. In a weird way, she felt as though this twenty-one-year-old girl had never arrived, as there was this confusing mismatch between the images of the twenty-one-year-old and the present forty-five-year-old daughter, although with her healthy mind, she understood of course that they were both one person.

I am purposefully using these dramatic examples, although I am sure that you have many of your own intense life moments, which you had put away into the deepest shelves of your memory, to make room for new (fresh) memories.

On a less dramatic scale, if you are a high-school student and you hate math, but do very well in English, you will tend to spend much more time writing essays because numbers and theorems make you feel distressed, and we know that everyone's EGO is looking for peace and balance. Things that aggravate your ID (your innermost desires), like diets, are very upsetting and uncomfortable for us, while things that make us happy take place comfortably and smoothly. You are simply living and enjoying your life.

I recall one of my patients who used to be a chain-smoker. I helped him quit smoking a long time ago and recently asked him if he is ever drawn to cigarettes. He remembers the smell of the cigarettes, he says, and even enjoys it, but he has not had a desire to smoke at all. And the image of his hand with the cigarette in it moving toward his mouth seems awkward and funny to him.

I think he is so comfortable because of the following:

- His ID enjoys the company of a friend smoking next to him.
- His SUPEREGO chooses not to smoke.
- His EGO is happy because it found balance between ID and SUPEREGO.

"The problem"—the issue of smoking—does not exist for this guy anymore.

We are slowly moving toward our ultimate goal in this book: to be able to lose unwanted weight naturally and to maintain it effortlessly.

CHAPTER 16

Are You Really Overweight?

I just want to make sure you are not playing mind games with yourself. Did someone call you fat, or do you think so yourself? As we have seen in the baby chapter earlier in the book (chapter 8), we are born balanced and beautiful.

You must have had your first encounter with the concept of "fat" early on in your life. The first-time experience creates a concept for you that had never existed before. Once the "known" is formed, though, you are often prompted to evaluate it using the moral and cultural standards, which the society is imposing on you. Let me clarify this seemingly confusing sentence.

If you were someone like me growing up in Ukraine in the '70s, I had no concept of gays, lesbians, and transgender people. Do I have your attention now? I had no opinion on this matter until I left Ukraine at age fifteen. I had no opinion on the matter and no feelings about this matter because the matter did not exist for me in the material world. Several weeks after I arrived in the United States, we were strolling in Greenwich Village in New York City and saw a couple of men walking down the street, holding hands. "Who are they?" I asked an alien question.

"Gay people" was the answer.

That day the concept of "gay" became material for me. Now, my brain would pick up on the five senses that would like antennae feel out the information regarding this matter in the media, print, on the streets, and so on, and my new brain would start processing this information under the heading "gay."

My daughter, on the other hand, was born here in New York City and was exposed to the concept of "gayness" when she was only eight years old, in her elementary public school. Her brain then became capable of processing all the info she started picking up on the matter from her family, her friends, her school, and her books to form a structured concept of what the word "gay" meant to her.

A black executive from Nigeria, who has been living in the United States since his early twenties, told me once, "The first thing I learned when I came to the United

States was that I was black. I did not realize it before that time."

The point is, once again, that unless a thought is brought into your awareness via any of the five senses (the more, the stronger), that concept does not exist either for your ID or for your SUPEREGO. The application of this concept has to do with pretty much everything you encounter in this life.

Have you ever thought about dieting as a child? Probably not. Most people are not aware of their excess weight until the moment someone has indoctrinated them in it. Someone has had to materialize this concept to their awareness. It may have been done loud and clear as one middle-school girl telling another in front of everyone, "You are fat!" Or it may have been done in a very subtle way as your young twenty-year-old boyfriend passing by and "lovingly" petting you on a shoulder, remarking, "Boy, you've gained weight, honey!"

One way or another the thought of you being over-weight was communicated to you using one or all of the five senses. At that moment, the concept of you in relation to your physical image was born, and the mind started actively tuning into the universe of data available to it on this subject.

What kind of information was your mind exposed to? Well, let's start with the TV and the movies. Roseanne Barr does not personify the image of beauty proposed to you by the society. Angelina Jolie personifies it. What do the dolls in the American Girl Place look like? Melissa McCarthy? No. They look like Sandra Bullock. The concept of skinny jeans and miniskirts does not work well with the Rubensian Women. It works for the tall and skinny model types. This is why the twentieth century has brought us more eating disorders, including anorexia, bulimia, and dare I say, being overweight? I totally understand that it's easier for famous clothing designers to drape their fabric on tall and skinny girls, but what does it have to do with us, regular people?

I am sure that there were fat cavewomen in prehistoric times, but the thing is they did not know they were fat. The thought was not materialized by their five senses, and the issue of dieting was nonexistent.

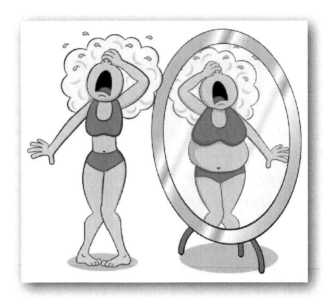

Of course, once you have realized that you are over-weight, the nasty conflict between the ID with its fondness for eating and the SUPEREGO with its quest for the beauty standard of the day began. As a result of this tug of war, you have been feeling anxious and insecure ever since. True, the discomfort is not as profound as it used to be because you are used to being overweight.

Have you ever seen a documentary about the first silent movies featuring steam locomotive moving at full speed toward the camera? These black and white documentaries show people in the "movie theater" getting very scared by the oncoming puffer. Some viewers are shielding their face, and some are outright running out of the movie theater. You know so much about the five senses, my friend, that this picture makes perfect sense to you, right?

The eyes of the viewers in the theater were transmitting the message: "a steam locomotive is speeding toward you." For someone who has never seen a movie before this would instantly be interpreted as a real danger by the brain, and the person would feel scared. A new "known" would be recorded for this person, and with repeated exposure to this type of a movie, featuring an oncoming locomotive, the mind would stop signaling danger. Eventually, there would not be any conflict between ID trying to feel comfortable and the SUPEREGO remembering its many safe exposures to the movie with locomotive. The result: people stopped being afraid of the movies featuring oncoming locomotives.

Imagine stepping on a water hose when it's pitch-dark all around you. I am chuckling because it actually happened to me more than once. The five senses are relaying to your brain that you are stepping on something long and moving on the ground. An instant decision is made—a snake! You feel anxious and withdraw your leg. You turn on the lights and see—a water hose! You feel calm and balanced again like this never happened, thanks to the fact that you know that water hoses don't sting with poison. It's a solid "known" that's been proven true many times before when you handled a water hose. But for one instance you felt how the other "known"—the snake—made you feel very scared. We could go on and on with endless examples of how SUPEREGO is looking for the most acceptable "known" because our life consists of an endless string of these situations, no matter where you turn.

Poor overworked SUPEREGO: if it finds the best decision it is looking for, then you feel content and balanced. However, if this decision does not sound acceptable to ID, then you become like a biochemical battlefield, with all sorts of negative emotions exploding all over you. Rest assured, your ID and SUPEREGO have not found their balance yet, my dear, because you have not been able yet to lose unwanted weight and maintain your ideal weight effortlessly. And so you may be unable to sleep well, or you may find yourself more aggressive than usual or very fatigued despite getting enough rest; this biochemical fight—this conflict between ID and SUPEREGO—has different effects on different people.

So, if you think you are truly over your ideal weight, at which you felt great and secure, and you are not just being forced into an image created by social media propaganda, read on.

CHAPTER 17

Recognize Your Critical Energy Switch

Most of you, folks, have something very important in common when it comes to weight loss. If I ask you how much you are eating, the majority would respond, "Doc, I hardly eat anything, and I still gain weight."

How do I know that you would say that? Because I treat people like you every day.

Imagine yourself as a car. In chapters 5 to 7, we have learned how the food we eat is turned into energy by our Cells. Your car needs energy, too. Let's say it's old-fashioned and runs on gas. The car has a little light that goes on when the gasoline level is decreasing. This does not mean that the car will stop right away. You will still be able to drive for another thirty to fifty miles, depending on the make of the car. After that your car will stop.

I have great news for you, folks: we humans have our own little switch, which also warns us when we are going to run out of energy soon. When I discovered the existence of this switch, so many things started making sense to me as a doctor. I called this built-in mechanism we have a CRITICAL ENERGY SWITCH.

In chapter 7, we spoke about how the body works to maintain energy necessary for our life functions. It turns out that it is our CRITICAL ENERGY SWITCH, which we are born with, that makes this monitoring possible.

The CRITICAL ENERGY SWITCH can only exist in one of the two positions: if it's turned OFF, we function in a Normal Mode. What does a Normal Mode mean? It means that whatever you just ate, is being used to produce the energy for living and functioning in the here and now.

When CRITICAL ENERGY SWITCH is turned ON, the body signals to us that we are "running out of gas"— that is, running out of energy. What happens then is that we enter the STARVATION MODE.

In the STARVATION MODE, your Cells are scared. They think, "Oh boy, who knows when is the next time our owner will feed us? Whatever he feeds us from now on, let's keep this stuff in storage bins, just in case. This will be our security blanket."

Some blanket! This is your fat, buddy!

If you don't eat every 3 to 3½ hours, the Critical Energy Switch will change its position from OFF to ON, and you will enter the Starvation Mode. So, please eat every 3 to 3½ hours, and you will avoid the Starvation Mode!

The body will sense that the food is abundant and available, so it will relax, and the balance will be achieved. Energy will be produced and used right away to power life functions, and nothing will be tucked away as fat.

How do you know that your body is going to run out of gas soon? In other words, how do you find out if the CRITICAL ENERGY SWITCH is ON?

Very simple: you feel HUNGRY! Hunger tells us, "Attention! I just switched your body into the STARVATION MODE. This is dangerous to your Cells, so they are going to start looking out for themselves. They will collect, store, and deposit into your fat bank all the food that comes their way, no matter what you eat from now on."

Let me give you a simple example.

Let's take my favorite dish: grilled fish and vegetables. If I eat it AFTER I felt hungry, a portion of it will be converted to fat, and I will gain weight. If I take the same dish and eat it BEFORE I get hungry, it will be used up for energy only, without fat production and weight gain.

So, how do we keep our CRITICAL ENERGY SWITCH in the OFF position? How do we avoid the STARVATION MODE? We should not wait until we are hungry! Hunger is like that little lamp in the car. It announces that you've already entered your STARVATION MODE. If you are feeling hungry, it is too late. You are already in the fat-producing mode.

The way to keep the CRITICAL ENERGY SWITCH in the OFF position is to supply the source of energy (good food) every 3 to 3½ hours.

Wait a minute!

Isn't that what the newborn baby did? In chapter 8—The Original Perfection—we talked about the baby's built-in eating clock. Guess what? Even though you may be older and taller, nothing changed in your old brain. You are still wired the same way—to eat approximately every 3 to 3½ hours.

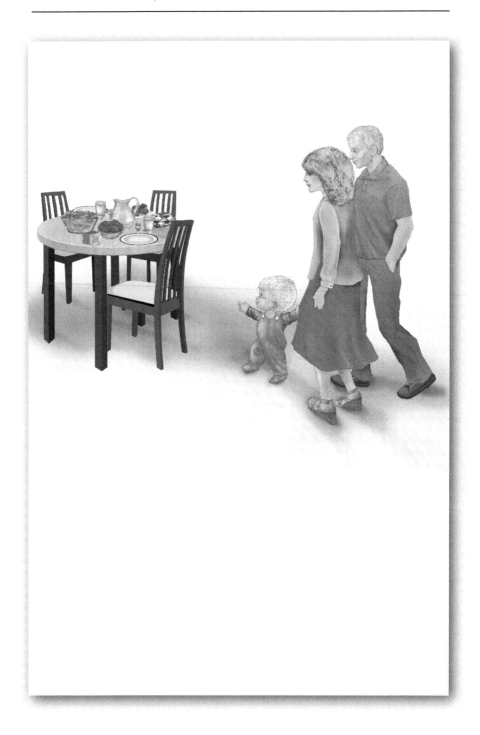

DIET SLAVE NO MORE!

Keep in mind that your CRITICAL ENERGY SWITCH does not negotiate. Once it is turned ᴏɴ and your body goes into the STARVATION MODE, it does not matter how much you will eat; the minimal amount of energy is allocated for survival, and the rest is stocked away in the fatty folds—your "security blankets." Actually, you can also think of yourself as a garbage bin at this point, since fat overloads your liver and disables it from doing its job properly.

Now you can understand why it's a big mistake to assume that if you eat only once a day, you should be losing weight.

Quite the opposite: eating once a day clearly gains you weight. Let's review why this happens:

1. The built-in timer (to eat every 3 to 3½ hours) becomes disrupted.
2. The CRITICAL ENERGY SWITCH gets turned ᴏɴ.
3. The body starts working in the STARVATION MODE.

147

4. Hunger prompts you to eat the amount of food much larger than the required regular norm, which was built into us. At this point you can't think straight and start making bad choices—you will eat anything.

5. Your stomach muscle is stretching from this excess of food because it is elastic and can stretch to accommodate our foolishness.

6. The stomach will remain perpetually stretched as a result of this repetitive pattern of living in the STARVATION MODE.

Your brain does not care if you are a neurosurgeon or a rocket scientist who does not have time to eat. It lives on the built-in schedule, which treats you the same way it treats your one-year-old grandson. Both you and your grandson will get the same signal to eat; the only difference is that you can keep delaying your meals, but he won't.

Let's take a snapshot of the day in the life of my overweight patient who lives in Connecticut and works in Manhattan as a computer programmer.

It is 1:00 p.m., and you have not eaten anything since stuffing yourself with a ham-and-cheese breakfast sandwich and coffee at 8:00 a.m. on your way to work. But you cannot afford going out to lunch, because you have a deadline to meet and your manager is already giving you the evil eye from his cubicle across the floor. Your colleague, Mindy, in the next cubicle is celebrating her son's graduation from high school and just brought in a box of donuts or cupcakes or chocolate-chip cookies or whatever, and you WILL have some; thank you. Continuing to chip away at your project. Shucks, why did I eat that? What's wrong with me?

It is 5:00 p.m. You are leaving work, having finished the project. "Next time, try to be more expeditious," your boss chides you on your way out. You still haven't had anything to eat. Riding on a subway, sullen, underappreciated, and hungry.

It is 6:30 p.m., assuming an unrealistically short commute. You just got home, and you are too tired to cook. You reach into your freezer for answers to your dilemma. The answers come in a shape of Bourbon Chicken from Costco, a frozen baked potato purchased months ago at a local supermarket, and a quart of salad from yesterday.

It's 7:00 p.m. You are putting away your dinner, while subconsciously you realize that you have gotten it all wrong again. You are upset and dissatisfied. You will start looking for another job tomorrow. Working for someone like your boss is a torture, and you've had enough. The frustration is somewhat relieved by the glass of wine or beer or whiskey or a joint, with your legs up on the table, while you start to watch the reruns of *The Real Housewives of...*

It's 9:00 p.m. The alcohol gives you a twinge of heartburn. You get up to put out the fire in your stomach with some pita chips with hummus or a bag of almonds or ice cream or whatever.

It's 10:00 p.m. You switch the channels. Stupid TV. You will have some tea. After all, it's herbal and is supposed to be good for you. You pour some tea with some sugar into a mug and feel like complementing your tea with a bite of something tasty, like a bit of peanut butter on whole-wheat bread—both are supposed to be good for you, right?

It's 11:00 p.m. The news. You are frustrated with the state of the world, but what do you matter in a grand scheme of things? You can't even impress your boss. You revisit the refrigerator. It contains many interesting possibilities for quelling what seems to be a permanent state of disenchantment with your life. You partake of some of them and watch a history channel—maybe you will finally learn something useful.

It's 11:55 p.m., and you have to go to sleep because tomorrow is another crazy day.

Revisit the idea of this chapter:

You were born with an eating clock built into your brain. Eat every 3 to 3½ hours to keep your Critical Energy Switch in the OFF position, to avoid triggering the Starvation Mode.

CHAPTER 18

Motivation in a Nutshell

Whether you are a working dad or a stay-at-home mom or a millennial with a pet, you are all facing the same dietary dilemma: you've been eating a certain way for years, and every attempt to deviate from that was temporary and resulted in more weight than before you went on a diet.

Let's quickly review why all diets fail:

- Dietary restrictions never work permanently because our Cells demand good food to produce energy properly, without dangerous wastes. (Chapter 7)
- Restrictions create the conflict between the ID and the SUPEREGO. (Chapter 14)
- Dietary restrictions contradict with our inborn eating clock. This clock makes sure that the CRITICAL

ENERGY SWITCH gets turned ON every 3 to
3½ hours, and the hungry body goes into the
STARVATION MODE, after which it is next to
impossible to lose weight permanently. (Chapter 17)

So, how do we not lose hope and make ourselves stick to
a good eating routine for a lifetime? After all, this routine
requires timely eating, portion control, and quality food—
all of which are clearly restrictions. Whoops! Are we in a
catch-22 situation?

Let's look at some situations and observe how ID and
SUPEREGO process them. Perhaps, we can find the road
to a solution this way.

You are relaxing on a couch after work in the evening.
There is a commercial break on TV, and they are advertis-
ing some yummy cookies, delicious and dripping with peanut butter or chocolate.

Five senses go to work:

- You are seeing these cookies.
- You go to the kitchen and smell whatever cookies or
  sweets you may have available.
- Your four-year-old son is asking, "May I have one?"

- You are tasting a piece and touching a cookie to check for freshness.

Isn't it amazing that even though you are just imagining all this, you are starting to feel a good, comfortable feeling? Some of you may even salivate at the thought of cookies. This, my dear, proves that your imagination is truly a sixth sense. But back to this weight-loss book:

- The neurons pick up on all of this information and bring it over to the brain for processing. (Remember the green envelopes in the picture with the neurons?)
- Your mind kicks in as well: the ID associates cookies with pleasure and initiates positive emotional reaction. You feel instantly comfortable.
- However, your SUPEREGO is considering this: "But we just had dinner. What kind of a pig am I?" Remember, only your SUPEREGO is capable of *analyzing* information received by five senses.
- It is the SUPEREGO that decides "to be or not to be."

The ID, however, is very primitive: it can only function like a switch with "+" position producing positive emotions and "–" position producing negative ones. Remember in chapter 13 we discussed how emotions were produced by biochemical reactions when neurons released miniature peptide molecules? Depending on what ID decides, these reactions will run in the positive or the negative direction, just like the urine dipstick pregnancy test would.

We get it why ID is so straightforward. After all it is associated with the older part of the brain, whose functions are limited to the following:

- **S**ex (procreation)
  and
- **P**leasure

Let's abbreviate these two functions as **SP**. These basic functions were super-important at the onset of human life on earth. Attacked by wild animals, natural disasters (volcanoes, floods, and earthquakes), and diseases, humans had to have a built-in mechanism guaranteeing survival of the species. Nowadays, the same two mechanisms help us survive one another. I have no idea who created this mechanism within us, but it has worked well for thousands of years, and here we are. Yeah!

Once again, your ID cannot reason or analyze. It can only receive something through five senses and categorize it as compatible with SP or not. ID receives information about the cookies and screens it against the SP criteria, looking for some compatibility. Yummy cookies are totally compatible with enjoyment in my opinion, on the basis of our "knowns" (unless you have fallen off the moon, where they have no cookies of course).

Click! ID initiates good emotions.

At the same time, your analytical SUPEREGO is thinking and choosing the proper course of action. The picky bastard is reasoning: "But I just had a dinner—let's skip the cookies. I want to be able to fit into that dress (or pants) I bought last week."

EGO delivers this decision to ID.

"What? No fun?" mumbles ID, and you feel instantly bad.

And this goes on and on. Every fraction of a moment, emotions can take a different turn depending on the situation and how ID feels about it. Imagine that you reluctantly cave in to your SUPEREGO and decide *not* to eat a cookie. You return to the couch to watch football (perhaps to make yourself feel a little better). Just as you have finished adjusting your reclining pillows and assumed a comfortable football-watching position, your four-year-old son comes up and asks, "Dad, can you help me find my crayons?"

Your irritated response: "Not now! Leave me alone!"

The boy's eyes instantly well up with tears, and he retreats into his room quietly. ID starts scanning for SP. Needless to say, there is no match. Click! ID initiates negative reactions, and you feel crappy.

At the same time, SUPEREGO is outraged at what is happening and intensifies this bad emotion, prompting you to get off your comfortable bed to walk over to your child to make amends. You feel horrible because you've upset your child for no reason. You then walk over to the refrigerator and make a peanut butter and jelly sandwich for both of you.

ID recognizes this: son does not cry anymore, and I am eating a delicious sandwich. This qualifies for SP, and you feel better.

However, SUPEREGO's verdict is this: "I am such a dufus. Why am I eating sweets after dinner?" A new conflict is born. You feel crappy again. And so it goes: ID initiates emotions, and SUPEREGO analyzes the same information received by five senses and decides what to do—what steps to take next. You can see that eating is just an example of how the same thing can make you feel two opposite emotions, like satisfaction and guilt. I am sure you have gazillions of examples from your everyday life when you have felt "conflicted" over something.

Does this mean that all eating plans are destined to fail? After all, unless they qualify for SP criteria imposed by your ID, these diets won't last for too long. We need some sort of motivation to make us stick with a healthy eating routine.

Let's continue to chip away at this dilemma. How do you motivate a person to do something?

Let's pretend that your three-year-old daughter is sitting on the floor playing with her doll. She is clearly enjoying herself. You all agree that playing with a doll qualifies for SP criteria.

You call out, "Jane, come here!"

No reaction.

"Come here, baby!"

Little Jane continues to play with her doll.

"If you come over, I will give you a present!"

Jane promptly gets off the floor and runs over to you. It's not that your daughter was ignoring you before. No, her SUPEREGO was simply making a choice to keep playing with her doll.

"Who knows why Mommy is calling me? Maybe to brush my teeth?"

But the new information about the present is a game changer.

"Maybe this present is more fun than the doll I am playing with," analyzes her SUPEREGO.

ID is matching a promised present with its SP requirements, and Jane runs over, happy with anticipation.

Hmm. It seems like we are getting somewhere. It appears that in order to deliberately agree to something and feel good about it, we need MOTIVATION.

Let's see if this works in another commonplace setting. It's 7:00 p.m., and you ask your teenage daughter, "Alex, why aren't you doing your homework?

"Leave me alone. I'm tired."

"If you study now, we can go see *Neighbors 2: Sorority Rising* tomorrow."

"Totally, Mom. I'm on it."

In both examples, with a three-year-old and with a teenager, the reward completely changed the children's behavior, while they felt great about making an effort.

OK. So we have MOTIVATION and REWARD, which helped us solve the problem of inertia. I didn't really get into the details of the movie, but you can see how it actually qualifies for both of the SP criteria imposed by ID and why SUPEREGO would easily agree to do the homework.

A reward creates motivation to do anything. Seriously, anything!

Consider a child who wants to become an Olympic or a world champion one day. What does it take to become one? From watching movies and talking to people, I imagine it takes an inhuman amount of painstaking training, which is far from fun and enjoyment. How is that possible? How do we make a child deliberately choose to go to a skating rink every day, for argument's sake, where they have to endure endless pain, falls, and fractures? Hello, this means bad emotions coming from ID! Won't SUPEREGO decide to quit, especially since the promise of the Olympic reward is so uncertain and is so far in the future?

I think it would take a very talented, and possibly a genius, coach to motivate a child to undergo these kinds of physical challenges. This motivation would have to fit at least one of the child's ID's SP criteria. Not only that: the rewards would have to change from time to time, as people get bored after a while, even with fun things. Indeed, it would take a combination of a very gifted child and an ingenious coach to keep up with the need for motivation needed to raise an Olympic champion.

I remember one renowned eighty-something-year-old musician, who told me that, in his entire life, he had only managed to raise one famous pianist—a winner of several international competitions and a popular performer. This elderly gentleman considered himself very fortunate to have found the "key" to his student's amazing drive to succeed.

It was thanks to exploring the subject of motivation that I have come to realize the need for some sort of an inspirational resource, which most people could relate to. This is how an idea was born for this book's companion—a Phone App called *Diet Slave No More!*

I wanted to make an app that would motivate you and reward you, so that you would keep working toward your weight-loss goal. And what better way to motivate someone than to introduce him or her to a friend or a partner?

CHAPTER 19

Meet Your Stomach

O K, so if we listen to our inborn eating clock, we should eat every 3 to 3½ hours, just before we start feeling hungry. But *how much* do we eat? Your *stomach* best answers this question. Take a look at the pictures here.

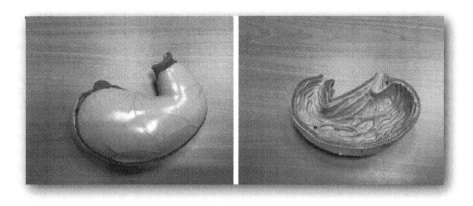

These photos are exact wax molds of the real human stomach. The one on the right is your stomach from the inside, and the one on the left is the same stomach from the outside.

When the human stomach is empty, it is as small as your hand and has the volume of approximately 180 to 240 grams, which is just about 6–8 oz.

Back in the anatomy class during my first year of medical school, I was amazed at how tiny the human stomach was in its empty state. After a full day of lectures and library studying, many of us came back to the anatomy lab by night to review the material. Legends about Michelangelo and Leonardo da Vinci sneaking into the morgue by night to study anatomy somehow made this boring duty more entertaining.

Of course, this being the late hours of the night, many of us would get hungry and eat our sandwiches right there in the anatomy lab, and the irony of this is striking me now, as the stomach I am referring to is winking at me from the depths of my memories.

The photo here illustrates that the stomach looks very much like the hand, both in its shape and size. I don't consider this resemblance a coincidence. Nothing in our amazing design is there by chance. I keep this model of the human stomach on the desk in my consultation room and always show it to weight-loss patients. They are amazed at how small it is! Our stomach was designed from a smooth muscle tissue, providing it with a capacity to stretch in case humans get a little too hungry. As we sit at the table in any diner or a restaurant in the United States, the portions we gulp down are enormous, and this poor little stomach just has to keep expanding.

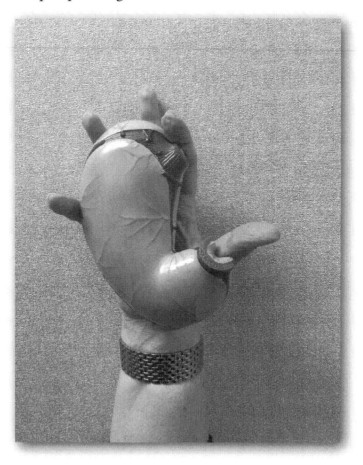

Imagine how your little stomach feels when it has to stretch so much. Organs remember things—it is a fact that was proven with the reports of people with transplanted organs experiencing new memories they never had before, but the deceased organ donors did. Every time you are taking your stomach out to a diner for a large meal, and every time you are putting away an entire pizza pie at home, rest assured that you are hurting your stomach's feelings.

People who go to the gym to work out know the feeling they get from sore, overworked muscles. Your stomach muscle also gives you that same bloated, burning, and achy feeling, after you have stretched it too much.

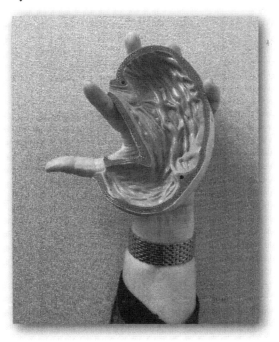

Looking at this photo of the inside of the stomach against the hand, I feel that Mother Nature came up with this design intentionally.

Perhaps, she wanted to bring your attention to the fact that a *portion of the meal necessary for your survival should fit into your hand!* She wanted you to have some kind of a guide, a measure; in case you were confused about how much is enough.

In fact, ancient Ayurvedic wisdom says that one should eat two handfuls size of a meal. If you consider how much fits into a handful, you will realize that two times that is approximately the size of your entire hand. So, the size of your hand is a pretty reliable visual representation of what the size of the meal on your plate should be.

"Oh no," you may passionately protest, "I eat much more than that!"

Yes, you are right. You have the capability to eat much more. Your stomach is made up of muscle tissue, which can stretch if it has to—that is, to make sure you don't die from your stomach bursting.

I recall watching a TV program recently, about some sausage-eating competition in the Midwest, and most recently in Brooklyn, New York, this past summer. Well, these guys' and girls' stomachs could really stretch!

Earlier in this book, we were "rewinding" our own life's movie backward, to the very infancy, and noted that the bottles bigger than 8 oz. did not exist. When you were first removed from your mama's watchful eye, to attend a daycare, or for some it was school, the portions grew out of control. College, work, and family just cemented the problem in place. I remember eating for hours at a time when I was an undergrad at Cornell. We had fun socializing and eating: food was a means of getting to pass pleasant time together. The pinnacle of our gluttony was eating heroes with meatballs at the legendary midnight truck on Stewart Avenue. I bet it's still there every night, surrounded by herds of hungry freshmen. And so it happened that year after year, while growing up, we were stretching our stomach's muscles. Endless social gatherings around the table, all-inclusive vacations, and eating marathons after work in front of TV would stretch it further.

Every one of you can rewind your own life's journey in your memory and try to analyze when exactly it was that your full stomach started getting stretched way beyond the size of your hand:

- Was it a gargantuan fast-food portion first introduced to you by the parent or a babysitter?
- Was it an evening out with the family at a local diner, serving portions that could knock out an elephant?
- Was it a college buffet with unlimited food over the discussion of philosophy or politics?

Or was it a giant steak you had eaten last night at a steak house, after attending to the contents of a bread basket and the tuna sashimi appetizer? Each one of us has his or her own gluttonous story, but all these roads lead to Rome—overstretching of our little stomach to the point where is starts looking like a pair of worn-out pantyhose.

Being a doctor makes me a sucker for an organized presentation of a concept. So, let me just summarize what, in my humble opinion, were the **three founding pillars**, supporting your original nutritional perfection, as a baby.

(1) **Your primary caretaker.** It was your mother or a grandmother or a babysitter or a stay-at-home father for some. All of them were extremely meticulous and loving when it came to preparing meals for you. A small piece of meat or poultry or fish, with some veggies, and maybe a small amount of potatoes or grains. This is what a smart nutritionist and a distinguished weight-loss expert would call "balanced meals."

(2) **Your eating schedule.** It essentially meant the exact times of the day that you were eating, as designated by your inborn eating clock, every 3 to 3½ hours.

(3) **Your eating portions.** That is your bottles, jars, and baby plates and cups, which your primary caretaker was using to feed you, the infant. These were never bigger than 8 oz., even for young toddlers. *The magic 8 oz.* never exceeded by your wise primary caretaker has an easy visual equivalent: *it is approximately the size of your hand!* And once again, if you lay your hand onto the wax model of your stomach, you will see the healthy natural size it was meant to be after a meal. What's important for our purposes here is that when you are going to eat your three meals and two snacks per day, the meal size should be about the size of

your hand, and the snack size should be about half of your hand.

I have some good news for you, big men and women: that ridiculously stretched-out stomach of yours still has a chance. If you eat small portions that fit the size of your hand and listen to your inborn eating clock, your stomach will start to shrink and, at some point, will get back to its original healthy size. What a wonderful, understanding muscle it is!

But are things really that simple? If everyone could just eat small portions every three hours, why would I be writing this book?

True, the stomach has no problem contracting back to its original size. The question is whether *you* could be disciplined enough to eat small portions of healthy balanced foods regularly. Could you?

If you compare your body design to your stomach's design, *you* are definitely more complex. You emerge from this comparison as an older brother, or a father figure. The stomach comes across as your younger sibling, your child, or your little friend. It is very kind and supportive. It will accommodate you by stretching or contracting—it's trying very hard.

A cool idea came to me when I started thinking about the Phone App: if our stomach friend could manage to do all these things to accommodate us, why couldn't we reciprocate and do something *to make him happy?* This is how the idea of an animated app character—Stomach Buddy—was born. Stomach Buddy becomes a partner, who motivates us to reach our weight-loss goals.

CHAPTER 20

Develop a New Eating Habit

T he moment has come when your patience is starting to pay off. On the basis of everything we have discussed so far, I am proposing the following steps with the goal of losing weight naturally and keeping it off forever. Here are the steps:

1. **Eat healthy food, which is good for your Cells.**
2. **Eat three meals the size of your stomach, which equals to the size of your hand and two snacks, the size of half of your hand.**
3. **Remember to eat every 3 to 3½ hours while awake.**

But how do we make these new eating routines stick? *How do we make eating healthy automatic?* Let's define automatic behavior. It is something that we do without thinking, because it satisfies our ID's SP requirements (sex or pleasure).

We all like to eat popcorn and drink soda at the movies. If you are someone who never felt this urge, you did not grow up in America as a child. This kind of behavior becomes automatic only when we are exposed to it many times over. Popcorn and soda at the movies have formed a strong synaptic web when they were processed by all five senses simultaneously and coupled with a pleasurable stimulus (a movie).

Automatic behaviors take place seamlessly and often without our conscious effort because they qualify for ID's SP criteria, like

- taking a shower,
- brushing our teeth,
- watching TV, and
- checking our e-mails.

If you start analyzing your behavior and tracing your steps back at the end of the day, you will come to a shocking realization that most of the things you have done during the day happened automatically, without conscious thought processing, as if you were living on an autopilot.

Imagine that you are driving home from work, down the same path every day. Most of the time, you are not even aware of how you got to your final destination—your home. The very first time you drove down that path from home to work and from work to home, you did it consciously of course. But after doing this repetitively for days, months, and years, you are driving on an autopilot, navigated by your subconscious. There is safety, familiarity, and a pleasure factor associated with the end of your working day, and you know that this qualifies for ID's SP criteria.

When I was doing my "on-call" shifts in medical residency, we worked about 80-85 hours per week. Every day you walked out of the hospital after 12-14 hours of work, still wearing your stinky scrubs, got home, took a shower, collapsed on your bed for 5 hours, and headed back to work, from Queens to Manhattan in my case.

I often wondered *how* it happened that I would take a number six train on Seventy-Seventh Street and Lexington Avenue, take it all the way down to Fifty-First Street, get off, change the platforms, and take an F or an E train going to Forest Hills, Queens. At the end of this commute (if there was any beginning or an end at this point), I had no recollection whatsoever of how I would get from point A to point B. Apparently, I had traveled in an automatic trance, without having my conscious brain participate. And yet, I have never fallen off the platform and never bumped into anyone or anything. Amazing!

I am sure each and every one of you has these stories of your own "hypnotic" travels from point A to point B, by foot or in a car. In this case, automatic brain activity gets you where you need to be and protects your life in the process.

Automatic behaviors can be very useful. Aren't you happy, for example, that your parents taught you to wash your hands after going to the bathroom?

Many of you may have developed a great automatic behavior of checking to see if your stove is turned off when you are leaving home. And I certainly hope that most of you will feed and walk your pets automatically, without ever forgetting, and remember to water your plants on time, and so on.

Closer to home, what we do after work, for example, is mostly automatic—especially since it's validated by ID's SP criteria:

- Sitting in front of TV and eating whatever.
- Reading and eating whatever.
- Smoking after eating a big meal.
- Eating when your friends or family are eating.
- Eating while checking e-mails.
- Kissing your children good night.
- Grabbing a beer or a glass of wine when you are in front of TV or computer.

We have already talked about the fact that it is impossible to erase an automatic behavior from your brain. Our brain is a repository of everything that has ever happened to us, especially if it happened repeatedly. Just in case you would ever need to access that memory. If you do not practice an automatic behavior for a while, it becomes a bit rusty but still exists there in the depths of your neuronal synapses, like an old painting in the museum storage, waiting to be exhibited.

Let's review steps 1–3:

1. Eat healthy food, which is good for your Cells.
2. Eat three meals the size of your stomach, which equals to the size of your hand, and two snacks, the size of half of your hand.
3. Remember to eat every 3 to 3½ hours while awake; All three steps **should be carried out in a pleasant setting many times over, in order to become our lifestyle—something we do automatically.**

Aristotle said, "We are what we repeatedly do. Excellence, then, is not an act, but a habit."

Habits become us. And the wise man lived so long ago that he was not even aware of building unbreakable synaptic webs. We are clearly better positioned to see why his statement makes sense.

And yes, let's make healthy eating fun! This way our ID will be satisfied and at peace with the SUPEREGO. Remember little James and his first pizza experience?

1. He saw it, surrounded by the happy kids.
2. He heard all the joyful squeals around it.
3. He smelled its delicious aroma.

4. He touched its warm crust.

5. He tasted its cheesy texture.

His first experience with pizza generated a strong positive "known" in his brain networks, approved by both ID and SUPEREGO.

The second ingredient in making the habit automatic is repetition. Repetition is by far the most powerful ingredient of habit formation known to the behavioral psychology.

Have you ever smoked?

I have. I used to smoke heavily in medical school, until one day I had an epiphany that I was being a hypocrite. How could I teach people to be good to their bodies if I was so rotten to my own? That was the day I quit smoking cold turkey, but few people are strong enough to do that. I am digressing, though, from the true reason I brought up smoking here.

I remember smoking my first cigarette. I was sitting in a balcony of my medical school's main building, with a bunch of fellow students. It was a warm spring afternoon, and the jokes and laughter were creating a warm and congenial atmosphere of bonding around us. My ID was reveling in pleasure—I was having fun! Even though the first puff of a cigarette offered to me tasted terrible and made me cough, I literally forced myself to smoke an entire cigarette. In those first rounds of repeating a behavior, like smoking, it is the social pressures that guide us. We do not even realize, in succumbing to those social pressures over and over again, that we are creating a habit beyond just one or two exposures to something we later realize is bad for us. Once again, thanks to the five senses, every object we have ever come in touch with repetitively becomes permanently recorded in our synaptic webs.

Realizing how profoundly strong these synaptic webs are can help us understand how we have been creating habits in our eating patterns. Remember I was referring to parents who were chatting with one another at the table in a restaurant, while their child was eating and watching a video? This was the beginning of a stimulus (food) coupled with a video (pleasurable setting) repetitively (I presume this was not the first or the tenth time this baby was watching a video while eating). For the rest of her life, this poor kid will have a "food" symbol light up in her brain when she turns on a TV set or a computer video.

If your parents rewarded you with candies for a good behavior or grades, you will have a memory of steel for that.

Our very language reinforces a strong association between sweets and feeling good: sweet loving, sweetheart, sweet deal, sweet life, and sweet Valentine.

Repetitive lifestyle patterns, which we choose to follow as adults, strengthen the synaptic connections between our routine and compromising eating habits. Take yourself, for example, when you come home after a full day at work. You have a dinner alone or with a spouse or a roommate or with the kids. This takes place at the table for some people, but for others it already takes place in front of TV. Have you even noticed how you got there with your plate?

Now, those of you who ate at the table, you probably cleaned up the dishes after dinner and, after some minutes or hours, would wind up in front of—that very TV or a computer. In a little while, the signal to eat will come over you automatically. You will get up, walk to the kitchen, and start munching on one of the following:

- Chips (organic or regular, baked, fried or whatever).
- Nuts (all kinds, roasted, toasted, salted, unsalted).
- Bars, crackers, pita (gluten-free or not).
- Cheese bites.
- Fruits.

- Chocolates, cookies, and candies.
- "Bites" of whatever else you bought in your supermarket from the "snack" isle.
- Wine (red or white) or hard alcohol.
- Coffee or tea with or without cream or milk or sugar.

This habitual snacking will last until you go to bed. No wonder you have trouble shedding those unwanted pounds despite sweating away in the gym every day of the week.

I am going to summarize this chapter by reviewing the **three steps I recommend for creating a new healthy eating habit:**

1. **Eat healthy food, which is good for your Cells.**
2. **Eat three meals the size of your stomach, which equals to the size of your hand, and two snacks, the size of half of your hand.**
3. **Eat every 3 to 3½ hours while awake.**

The following "formula" summarizes how to turn steps 1–3 into an automatic habit:

New Eating Habit = Steps 1–3 + FUN + Repetition.

Initially I felt very tortured about where to get the FUN ingredient, which is essential for this formula to work. Could our sixth sense—our imagination—fill in this gap?

"Everything you can imagine is real," said Pablo Picasso, and I agree. Let's play a game to illustrate this concept.

Close your eyes and imagine yourself with your significant other, on a beautiful summer night, sitting on a bench, under the stars and the moon, with a bottle of champagne and some cheese. Write down how you feel.

Just so you know that I am with you on this journey, I just did this myself, and the feeling I produced was that of a loving excitement.

Now, I want you to close your eyes again and keep the same context: "yourself with your significant other, on a beautiful summer night, sitting under the stars and the moon, with a bottle of champagne and some cheese." But add a new detail: you are not on a bench but instead perched on a huge jungle-tree branch.

Dwell on what emotion this mental visualization produced. (Mine was anxiety, since I felt as though there was a snake or some other jungle-night creature that was staring at us from the darkness.)

Let's close our eyes again and visualize the same context: "yourself with your significant other, on a beautiful summer night, under the stars and the moon, with a bottle of champagne and some cheese." This time, replace the detail of a jungle-tree branch with the Garden of Eden.

Note your emotion. (Mine was that of a peaceful bliss.) Yet again, close your eyes and imagine or visualize the same context: "yourself with your significant other, on a beautiful summer night, under the stars and the moon, with a bottle of champagne and some cheese." But this time replace the detail of Garden of Eden with a cave where a huge tiger dwells.

Make a note of how you feel. (My emotion is that of pure horror.)

Now, let's adjust the imagery a little bit by chaining the tiger to the wall.

Close your eyes and visualize the same familiar context, but with the new detail of a chained tiger, baring his fangs at you and roaring.

How do you feel? (I feel fear but not the worst kind. Just hope that chain is strong enough.)

All right. I know you are tired. Relax. Do you see where I am going with all of this? If you don't, that's perfectly fine, since for most of us the concept of mental exercise is a new one. In the past several minutes, by manipulating the details of a context, you managed to sequentially create several very different emotions. Isn't that amazing? So originally I was hoping that the folks reading this book would just bring themselves to having a good time while preparing their meals or getting ready to eat them. Like when eating a salad, I often recall how I handpicked every vegetable, how wonderful it tastes, and how excited my Cells are to partake of this goodness. But I learned that for most people, mental exercise is tiring and confusing, and therefore NOT FUN for their ID.

So, exciting yourself into feeling happy was a no-go area for my self-help book. I had to come up with something EVERYONE could use effortlessly, so that their ID would be satisfied. And this is where my app came to the rescue. *Diet Slave No More!* Phone App has this cute little stomach character, which speaks and sings in a child's voice. Stomach Buddy motivates my readers to carry out steps 1–3 from this chapter every day and makes it fun in the process!

CHAPTER 21

How Long Does It Take?

I often get asked how long does it take to "wire in" a new habit or an automatic behavior? On the basis of my clinical experience and inspired by the esoteric literature I have analyzed, I have arrived at *forty days* as the answer. That's how long it takes to create a new healthy eating lifestyle.

The meaning of this number could be purely coincidental to my clinical experience, but there is a strong possibility for a more symbolic significance. For example:

- Moses spent forty days and forty nights on Mount Sinai communicating with G-d.
- According to gospels, Jesus fasted in the desert for forty days, tempted by Satan.

- In many cultures, folk wisdom upholds that to recover from delivering a child, a woman needs forty days. It may take this long for the energies of the mother and a child to reorganize themselves, to find their independent balance.
- The book of Genesis says that it rained for forty days and forty nights when G-d wanted to cleanse the Earth and start all over.

What is the significance of all these stories for our book? It means that we need to add step 4 to our new routine:

1. **Eat healthy food, which is good for your Cells.**
2. **Eat three meals the size of your stomach, which equals to the size of your hand, and two snacks, the size of half of your hand.**
3. **Eat every 3 to 3½ hours while awake.**
4. **Repeat steps 1–3 for at least forty days in a row.**

Of course, the best way to create a strong new routine is to make that forty-day exposure very rewarding, which first of all means being nonrestrictive as far as what you are eating. Removing the "forbidden fruit" element from the diet allows for a balance between your ID and SUPEREGO, instead of a conflict between the two.

As I have mentioned before, it's best to eat your small healthy meals in full awareness, without interference from TV, computer, or books. This is not a waste of your time. This is your cellular nourishment time. And trust me—it takes very little time to eat this food, which you can bring to work with you in small, apportioned containers.

Complete your forty days of continuous initiation of the new habit. At the end of this time frame, your mind and a happily shrunk stomach will be ready for occasional exceptions, like restaurant dates, holiday dinners with the family, and vacations. The most wonderful thing is that your mind, previously conflicted between ID and SUPEREGO, will now have reclaimed its eating comfort zone. After the forty days of eating healthy, eating out will never compromise you anymore. Your body will just be asking for what you are newly used to. No more and no less. And by the way, if you love your children and your family, wouldn't it be nice to let them in on your new and satisfying way of nourishment? Perhaps they would benefit from it, too?

After your forty days are done, try to stick to your new healthy eating habit at least six days per week. Everyday food should be like everyday clothing (clean and simple): fresh, natural, and balanced. However, we all own clothing and jewelry meant for celebrations (fancy), and that is where your one day per week allocated for eating out fits in. Eating out should be a special occasion. And if you do eat out, you can eat whatever you wish, but keeping in mind the size of your stomach—the size of your hand.

CHAPTER 22

The Missing Link

About three years ago, I had finished writing the first seventeen chapters of the book, and then I stopped and reassessed my work. I was satisfied with the way the book explained why we eat and why good food is important for our Cells. I was also excited about sharing with you the workings of our brain—how it processes information around us, how our emotions are manufactured, and what makes us vulnerable to brainwashing. At that point I had formulated the three steps that had to be carried out for at least forty days in order to become your healthy eating lifestyle forever.

But something was missing…

In my clinical practice, I noticed that while some patients who were following my "prescription" were losing weight and maintaining the weight lost, there were also other patients who had never succeeded to lose any significant amount of weight.

I started analyzing routines of those folks who had failed to lose any weight. Among them were some who forgot to prepare their meals the day before and just ran out of the house in the morning, having eaten a random breakfast, a random lunch at a random time, from a random nearby food truck or café. These patients had gotten a detailed plan from me on how to do it, but they just did not have the time or the stamina to implement the plan. There were also other patients, who did prepare their meals and prepackaged them for work the day before, but forgot to eat them at appropriate times during the day.

Overall, it was hard for people to recreate the three founding pillars of their original nutritional perfection; namely, their primary caretaker (someone to cook properly), their eating schedule, and eating portions.

Some folks just never cooked in their life and were lost. For those I recommended fresh-food-delivery services, which would cook and deliver three apportioned meals and two snacks to their clients' doorstep every morning. While this had worked for some patients, there were many issues with fresh-food-delivery services. They were too expensive for most people, and the meal choices were often limited and rarely organic or non-GMO (genetically modified organisms).

Then there were also some women patients who loved to cook and hated the idea of someone cooking for them. However, they were so used to huge portions at random eating times that they just could not get over these stumbling stones. I tried to convince these ladies that there was something liberating in having someone cook for them for a little while and that, at the very least, they could spend less of their precious time on shopping for food and cooking it, and anything else that had to do with this process (driving or walking to the market, unpacking, washing, cooking, cleaning, etc). Shopping at the big supermarkets and large wholesale distributors was also very tricky for these patients. They would emerge from their shopping with full bags of what? Plenty of unhealthy snacks to have around the house to compromise their eating habits.

Overall, I found that preparing five containers filled with healthy nutritious food (three small ones for meals and two tiny ones for snacks) the night before was very important for succeeding. But how come some people managed to always prepare their little containers with food and others did not?

Yes. Something was clearly missing from my healthy eating plan. It had to work for everyone, not just for selected supermotivated and superorganized people.

For three years, I was painstakingly searching for a way to reach out to my patients at home, when they are at their most vulnerable, and to encourage them not to give up on their efforts. Here was my problem in a nutshell:

- Patients did not stick with their inborn eating clock and forgot to eat every 3 to 3½ hours.
- Patients forgot that the size of their meal should not have exceeded the size of their hand.
- Patients would lose motivation quickly, unless they maintained frequent follow-ups where I would inspire them over and over again.

Of course, the SUPEREGO part of their mind was thinking, "You are fat. It is time to listen to Dr. Kogan and do what she tells you to do. Otherwise you will be unhealthy, depressed, and unable to fit into your clothes, blah, blah, blah." However, this was always at odds with their ID's simple outlook on life. Steps 1–3 did not fit ID's SP criteria (sex or pleasure). As a result, there was a conflict between ID and SUPEREGO, and that was an ultimate problem for this weight-loss plan.

Alcoholics know that they are destroying their life and the life of their loved ones, and they know what the right thing to do is, but just cannot stay away from drinking alcohol. Unless—they become members of Alcoholic Anonymous or a similar organization and get assigned a Sponsor, who guides them and protects them from their ID. Eureka!

My plan needed a "Sponsor"! Its main functions were designated as follows:

- Remind my patients to eat every 3 to 3½ hours.
- Remind them of how small their stomach is.
- Motivate them to stick with the plan, by making it fun for their ID.

Essentially, the Sponsor would be like our mind's EGO—helping to establish a balance between our pleasure-seeking ID and analytical SUPEREGO.

Of course, I was already serving as an EGO figure to many private patients, who had my cell-phone number and my e-mail address, and had access to me whenever they had cravings or lost their inspiration. They were the ones who were succeeding with their weight loss way ahead of everyone else! But how many people could I physically serve in my spare time, which I had very little of? And there were so many folks, who could not afford having me as their EGO buddy.

What if I came up with a Phone App, which anyone could afford and have it with them anytime and anyplace?

Great idea! An app was a doorway to meeting a friend who would look out for your interests. Amazingly, you would also feel like taking care of your buddy. I read a study that found that altruistic actions, like when you helped someone out, increased the release of oxytocin and dopamine—satisfaction molecules.

Since this book felt like my child after so many years in the making, the app felt like a grandchild. Naturally, it had to bear its mother's name—Diet Slave No More! My "grandchild" app introduces you to your impersonated stomach (Stomach Buddy). Initially, he is very sad because of what had been done to him over the course of his life.

He looks like this.

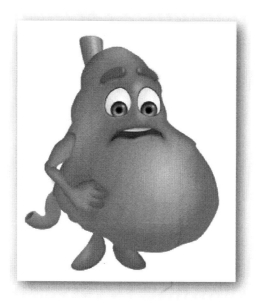

He is a very dreamy creature who reflects wistfully on what he looked like originally, when he was young and treated well by you.

Back in those good old days, you see, he looked like the stomach on the next page.

Your stomach character is an awesome buddy! He works for you around the clock, reminds you to eat, analyzes your weight change, praises you for succeeding to lose weight, and inspires you to get up and try again when you fail.

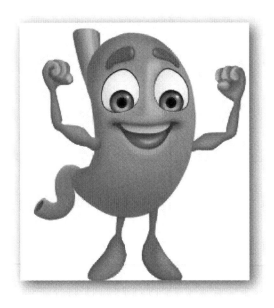

Your new little stomach friend makes you want to take care of him! Oxytocin related or not, we all have it in us to help someone in need. Even the worst of us will lend a helping hand to those in trouble. I knew a very mean lady who cared for no one. But on 9/11, even she was out there in downtown Manhattan, giving out donuts to firemen and policemen who were working through the rubble.

Once the missing link was identified and plugged in, I realized that my book was now complete and ready to be printed. Because now I would not just be sharing my "know how" with the world, but I would also be helping people for real. Helping them to reconcile the ever-present conflict between their inborn tendencies to indulge and to make things right.

Having read this book and downloaded the Diet Slave No More! app, you are now well positioned to make all four steps necessary to return to your Original Nutritional Perfection:

1. **Eat healthy food, which is good for your Cells.**
2. **Eat three meals the size of your stomach, which equals to the size of your hand, and two snacks, the size of half of your hand.**
3. **Eat every 3 to 3½ hours while awake.**
4. **Repeat steps 1–3 for at least forty days in a row.**

You have a shoulder to fall back upon—a supportive buddy who will watch over you and motivate you to simply do what you need to do to feel happy and balanced again.

CHAPTER 23

I Have a Dream

We are at the end of our literary journey. You understand now what needs to be done so that you can feed your Cells well and get back to your Original Perfection. Just to recap, new healthy eating habits can be developed by sticking to the following steps:

1. **Eat healthy food, which is good for your Cells.**
2. **Eat three meals the size of your stomach, which equals to the size of your hand, and two snacks, the size of half of your hand.**
3. **Eat every 3 to 3½ hours while awake.**
4. **Repeat steps 1–3 for at least forty days in a row.**

It is only by coming to understand what makes you who you are and what is the meaning of the food you eat that you can experience the "Aha!" and the desire to undergo forty days of eating the right way, to incorporate this healthy way of cellular nourishment into your lifestyle permanently.

Before you move on to this book's companion app, I invite you to take a fun quiz to determine whether this app will help you on your quest.

Let's Have Fun Quiz

Please answer the following questions with a "Yes" or "No" response:

1. Would you want to help an adult person who is not doing well?
2. Would you be inclined to help out an adult person who feels great?
3. Would you like to help a child who is not doing well?
4. Would you be inclined to help a child who feels great?
5. As a child, did you ever like cartoons?
6. As an adult, do you still like cartoons?
7. Do you like music?
8. Do you like to sing when no one can hear you?
9. Do you enjoy contributing to charity?
10. Do you enjoy giving presents?
11. Do you enjoy receiving presents?
12. Do you ever think about your childhood?
13. Has anyone ever sung you a lullaby?
14. Has anyone ever read a book or told you a goodnight story at bedtime?

15. Do you remember what kind of food you ate as a child?

16. Do you remember favorite smells from your childhood? (cooking, perfumes, etc.)

17. Do you remember kids from your elementary school?

18. Do you enjoy your childhood memories?

19. Do you like to be inspired and motivated to get things done?

20. Do you like loyalty?

21. Do you appreciate a good friend?

- If you answered at least 50 percent of the questions with a "Yes," I highly recommend that you buy my Phone App.

- If you answered at least 75 percent of the questions with a "Yes," you ought to own this app.

- If you answered 95–100 percent of the questions with a "Yes," getting this app is sacred and meant to be.

- If you answered 25 percent of the questions with a "Yes," you should still get this app.

- If you answered all the questions with a "No," your chances of getting this app are close to a zero. However, I think you will still want to get it, out of sheer curiosity.

It's likely that even you will find this app fun and helpful. Your age and sex do not matter. You just have to own a cell phone.

I have a dream that everyone who reads this book and downloads the app, will be able to return to his or her Original Nutritional Perfection effortlessly and forever. Here is to you, dear reader, and to your happy return to yourself!

APPENDIX 1

Boring Stuff (about Proteins, Fats, and Carbohydrates)

A. Proteins

You could not exist without proteins. They make up your Cells and are the key players in messaging, signaling, transportation, and DNA replication—all the vital cellular functions. By now you should be used to the fact that everything in life is made up of smaller stuff. So, it probably comes as no surprise that proteins are also made up of smaller building blocks called "amino acids." We make some of these amino acids on our own in the liver, but there are nine special amino acids, called "essential," which we cannot manufacture. We must import them from the food we eat. Without these essential amino acids, proteins cannot do their job properly.

Some people even buy these essential amino acids as supplements, but you don't have to. You can get essential amino acids from healthy balanced meals, even if you are vegetarian. You can google "where do essential amino acids come from in food" for some awesome resources, but for the purposes of our book, let's keep it simple. You should know that some protein comes from vegetables and grains but most comes from nuts and seeds, meats, fish, legumes, eggs, and dairy products, like milk, yogurt, or kefir.

How much protein do our Cells need? About 20–30 percent of your diet, but really it depends on how physically active you are. If you are a very sedentary woman or man who does not work out at all, you will need much less than a very physically active person or an athlete. It's just common sense. I am not feeding any numbers to you—you have all seen them and got nowhere with your calculations.

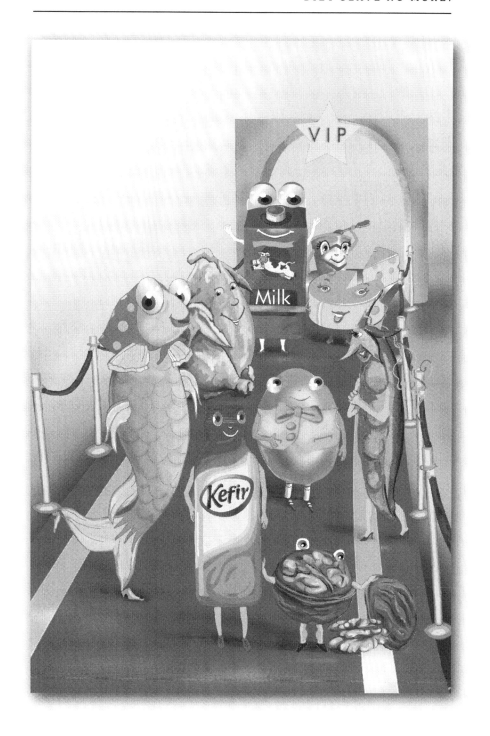

If your food is deficient in protein, which can sometimes happen if you are a vegan who does not know how to cook, or if you are recovering from a serious surgery, your body will start breaking down your own muscle and other structural tissues to manufacture proteins on its own. You can imagine an emaciated child from Africa as an extreme example of this horrible deficiency. But even on a less dramatic scale, if our diet is even somewhat deficient in protein, our immune system starts malfunctioning, hair and nails get brittle and the list of health issues gets longer.

At the same time, I hate to see some people *over*loading their body with protein, through shakes and powders. Most people do not benefit from too much protein, except professional athletes. But even athletes can develop fatal kidney conditions, related to chronic protein overload.

B. Fats

Well, just like you cannot exist without proteins, you cannot live without fats either. Like proteins, fats also make up your Cells. They are also involved in your immune system, hormone production, brain health, digestion, and vitamin absorption.

Just like with proteins, we can make most fats on our own in the liver, but we cannot make some special fats, and they must be uniquely imported from our food. These essential types of fats are found in the highest amounts in nuts, seeds, and fish.

If you are a vegetarian, use google to search "where do I get my essential fats from food" for the details. For the purposes of this book though, I just want you to have an understanding of why your Cells care about good food versus bad food. And that's why I want to talk to you about good fat and bad fat.

Unsaturated Fats versus Saturated Fats

How to make sense of this?

If you live in a well-built home or apartment, which can withstand storms and earthquakes, it makes you feel secure, doesn't it?

Well, the thing that makes your Cell feel secure is its home, called Cellular Membrane.

In fact, in addition to being Cell's home, a healthy Cellular Membrane is like a great country for the Cell to live in: it is keeping the Cell strong and independent, importing and exporting the goods, and keeping its cellular citizens and surrounding Cells happy.

Well, there are fats, which make Cellular Membranes/homes healthier and more efficient—they are called **unsaturated fats**. In kids, these unsaturated fats are also required for a healthy Nervous System development. You can do a google search for "where do I find unsaturated fats in food," but for the purposes of this book, just know that foods rich in unsaturated fats include nuts and seeds, avocadoes, coconut and olive oils, and fatty fish like salmon.

For every good guy, there always exist a couple of villains. C'est la vie! The home breakers, who destroy Cellular

Membrane and make you age faster and sicker, are called **saturated and trans fats**. Where do they come from?

Mostly from red meat, butter, lard, ice cream, and cheese, to mention a few. Saturated fat can be eaten in very small amounts. **But most of your fat intake should come from unsaturated fat.** It helps to remember that something like ice cream is not a dessert, or an after meal. It's a full meal. If you are not a diabetic, you can occasionally have one—if you so desire. About 20–30 percent of your diet should come from fat. The amount really depends on how healthy and active you are. Also, if you have issues with cholesterol and heart, try to opt for the plant-based sources of fat, which are cholesterol-free. Once again: common sense, folks—I am not here with numbers and tables. Been there, done that. Don't get fixated on numbers. The important thing to understand is that our Cells really care about what you are feeding to them.

C. Carbohydrates

These "guys" are the *easiest* to use for energy by the Cell and therefore comprise the biggest portion of our diet: about 40–60 percent. In layman's language, people call them "sugars." In this book, I have used both "carbohydrates" and "sugars" interchangeably.

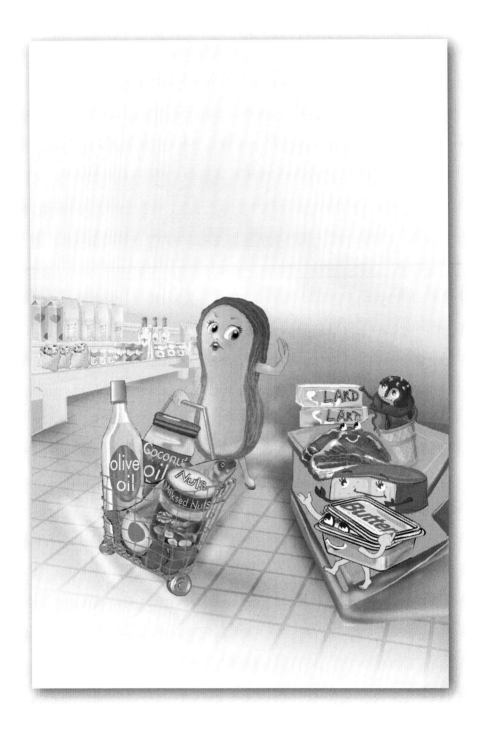

What's important for us to know is that liver is the boss of sugar regulation. Liver is like a sugar policeman who is aware of all the carbohydrates entering the body. He regulates: "this goes here, and this goes there."

This "policeman's" job is to keep blood-sugar levels healthy and to supply enough to the Cells so that they can make energy out of it. One common sugar used to make energy is called "glucose." Liver "policeman" is always watching glucose levels, and if they fall too low for some time, he starts making sugar out of proteins or fats.

The recommended daily allowance for total carbohydrates is 40–60 percent of your total daily food intake, depending on how healthy and active you are. However, keep in mind that it is not the carbohydrates in and of themselves that make us fat. It is the excess calories, which they provide when we tend to overeat them as we do very often. Too much food of any kind, whether it is rich in fat, protein, or carbohydrates, will gain you extra weight. Once again, don't get bogged down with the numbers and calories.

Another question that patients often ask me is this: Which carbohydrates/sugars are good and which are bad for your Cells? In order to answer this question, let us briefly discuss the two important categories of sugars.

Simple Carbohydrates versus Complex Ones

You cannot imagine how many times I revised the last two chapters over the last three years! Initially, they sounded like a biochemistry textbook, and I just kept simplifying and simplifying. I felt somehow that the reader should be able to understand and connect with what is happening inside the body, on a childlike and almost symbolic level. I digress—back to *simple* sugars.

On the surface these simple carbohydrate "guys" look so yummy: pastry, candy, cookies, ice cream, and soda, to name a few. They are rather simple for the body to digest and get absorbed into the blood very *quickly*. And that is very bad news for us. The quicker the sugar comes into the blood, the more the havoc it wreaks in the liver and blood.

As simple sugars rapidly enter our bloodstream, the liver "policeman" calls upon his partner pancreas to release a "police dog"—a hormone called *insulin*—and together they all go to work, trying to clear "the streets" of blood vessels from all that sugar floating in there.

Imagine insulin doggies running around desperately trying to secure wild sugar villains into handcuffs. In reality, insulin is desperately trying to move extra sugar into the tissues (muscle and the liver itself), but if you can imagine insulin handcuffing the sugar, you will do just fine.

In the meantime, nasty simple sugar characters are doing the damage all around them: they are gluing proteins to one another making them dysfunctional. This process, called "cross-linking" in medical-research slang, causes plaques in the arteries, cataracts, kidney disease, and many more awful things. As a matter of fact, as a high-school student, I became a Westinghouse national science competition semi-finalist for my research on protein cross-linking in the eyes of diabetics.

Now, complex carbohydrates represented by vegetables, beans, and grains, are the good guys. They are bigger molecules, and we digest them slowly. As a result, they enter our bloodstream gently and politely. The liver "policeman" and his fellow pancreas are happy to see complex sugars. Sure they are still subject to convoy but on much nicer terms. A few insulin "doggies" are slowly coming out sniffing these sugars and walking them out of the bloodstream into the tissue Cells, where they will be put to work to make energy for the body.

An additional perk of complex carbohydrates is that they are "dressed" in fiber, which behaves like an Oscar outfit: a long gown and stilettos; it slows down your entry into the ballroom of bloodstream. And that is a wonderful thing, to come into our bloodstream slowly and politely. Thank you, Mrs. Fiber!

"What about fruits?" asks my sweet-toothed reader. "Dr. Kogan, you are telling me that the bakery isle is off limits for me, but can I indulge in eating sweet fruits?"

I sadly report to you, dear reader, that fruits are not so innocent, as they are composed mostly of fructose, which is a simple sugar. That is why downing *a lot* of fruits is not going to be healthy for you. However, a beautiful thing about fruits is that most of them have lots of fiber, which makes them behave kind of like a complex carbohydrate.

Fruits should absolutely be a staple of your daily diet, as they are chock-full of vitamins, but if you are an older person or someone sedentary or someone simply trying to lose excess weight, keep those fruit portions small.

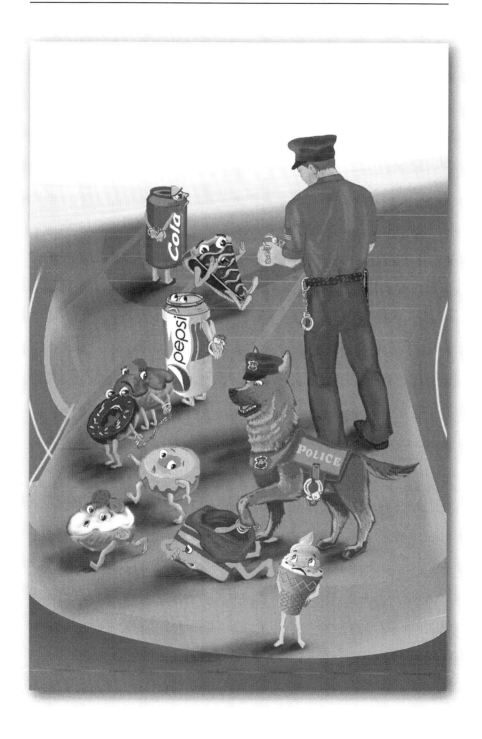

Also, keep in mind that if you drink fruit juice instead of eating fresh fruit, you are shutting out our wonderful Mrs. Fiber. Without her, sugars rise in the bloodstream too fast, harming everyone around them. You can tell I am not very fond of juicing.

Another thing to keep in mind when it comes to the simple versus complex carbohydrates concept is that all processed food has simple carbohydrates and all fresh veggies, beans, and grains have complex carbohydrates. So, stay away from processed food, which ironically means staying away from 95 percent of foods in your supermarket.

High Glycemic Index Carbohydrates versus Low Glycemic Index Carbohydrates

If the complex versus simple carbohydrates concept measures *"how fast* your blood sugar goes up when you eat a given carbohydrate," the concept of glycemic index measures *"how high* your sugar goes up after you eat something with carbohydrate in it."

You now understand just how important this is.

The higher the glycemic index, the worse is the carbohydrate and vice versa.

Classically, everything gets compared to the villainous white sugar, which has a glycemic index of one hundred.

What are some common examples of foods with a high glycemic index?

- White bread
- White rice
- Corn flakes
- Cookies
- Most processed snack foods

This is a much-abbreviated list. Ninety-five percent of your supermarket shelves are loaded with things with a high glycemic index, and these foods are to be avoided as much as possible.

I often get asked about what fruits are the safest to eat, and that's when I like to turn to the glycemic index. So, for example, if you are looking for low-glycemic-index fruits, which will be entering blood stream slowly and politely, go for apples, peaches, cherries, grapefruit, pears, plums, strawberries, blueberries, raspberries, and blackberries.

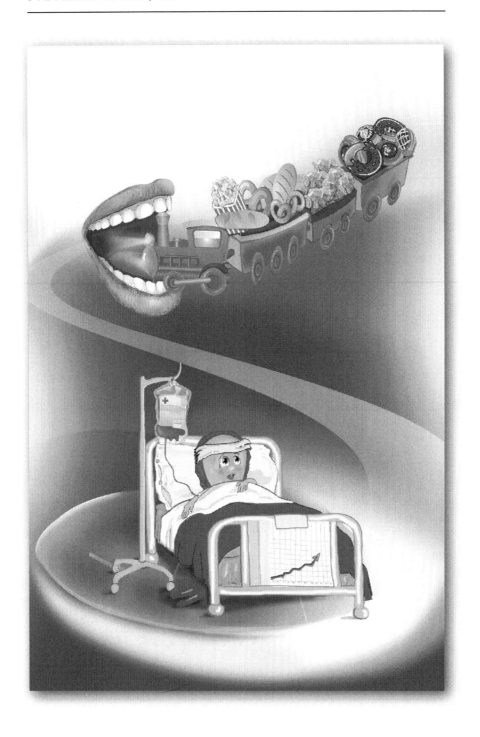

What are the high-glycemic-index fruits to stay away from if you are trying to lose weight? They are watermelon, raisins, pineapple, oranges, bananas, and any fruit juice because of the absence of Mrs. Fiber in the juices. The take-home message for you, dear reader, is that the majority of your daily carbohydrate intake should come from the lower-glycemic-index, higher-fiber, complex-carbohydrate foods, especially so if you are diabetic or prediabetic.

Now, what was the point of talking about all these fats, proteins, and carbohydrates (sugars)?

To understand what enters the Cell.

Chapter 6 reveals what happens to this entire tiny foodstuff inside the Cell.

APPENDIX 2

Good-Food Tips

Needless to say that you are eager to eat the kind of food that is healthy for your Cells. Here are some of my tips for keeping it real.

1. If possible, try to buy organic food or at least non-GMO

Organic farmers abide by very strict regulations, which forbid them to use synthetic pesticides (insecticides and herbicides) and chemical fertilizers for their crops. Why do we care? Well, pesticides are designed to kill, and because their mode of action is not specific to any particular species, they are killing us too. In most cases, they are killing us slowly, causing toxic side effects on our Digestive System, resulting in unexplainable abdominal symptoms and airway spasms, which in turn results in more asthma attacks in our population.

Organic meat and milk farmers do not use cancer-inducing hormones and stay away from antibiotic use. Toxic by-products of antibiotics fed to livestock can get transmitted to us, causing yeast infections and diarrheas and upsetting the natural flora of our intestines. I hope a day will come when organic food will become the standard of farming and will become affordable to everyone. Until then, at least try to look for more affordable non-GMOs produce.

GMO crops has plants' DNA altered to yield larger, more profitable crops. Why do we care? Because GMO foods have been found to cause many diseases in animals, and many suspect that GMO foods are related to the increasing incidence of asthma cases in the United States. At the time this book is being written, there are eight crops from GMO seeds produced in the United States:

- Corn
- Soybeans
- Cottonseed
- Canola
- Alfalfa
- Sugar beets

- Papaya
- Squash

Food labeled "USDA Organic" is automatically non-GMO by definition, but it is significantly more expensive than food labeled just "Non-GMO." See what you can afford, but at the very least, be mindful of the following twelve foods, which the research by Environmental Working Group has found to contain extremely high levels of pesticide residues. If nothing else, buy *these* organic! At the time this book is being written, here is the "dirty dozen," in order from most toxic to least toxic:

- Apple
- Strawberries
- Grapes
- Celery
- Peaches
- Spinach
- Sweet bell peppers
- Nectarines
- Cucumbers
- Cherry tomatoes

- Snap peas
- Potatoes

2. Avoid using any artificial sweeteners

Avoid artificial sweeteners such as Splenda (sucralose), SweetN'Low (saccharin), Equal and NutraSweet (aspartame). In my opinion, all of them are carcinogenic. By not drinking any soda and by not buying any sugar-free foods, you can assure yourself that you are not getting any of this poison in your blood. What would I recommend to sweeten your coffee, tea, or desserts? For a daily use, I would recommend stevia, which is plant derived, safe, and has almost no calories. For occasional indulgences, I use organic honey or organic brown sugar, or organic agave syrup. For diabetics, I recommend only stevia, xylitol, or honey as sweeteners, because of lower glycemic indices of these products.

3. Favor *fresh* fish

Source your fish from local small or big specialized seafood businesses, which ship fresh seafood daily or offer a catch of the day. The person cleaning your fish at the store should be able to identify the names of the fish, where it was caught, and whether it comes from freshwater or saltwater source. I do not believe in fish being organic—it is a selling gimmick. Just buy wild caught fish, not farmed. Farmed fish has many issues, which are beyond the scope of this book. I consider wild caught fish to be organic by definition—untouched by humans in their native habitat.

Fresh fish should not smell fishy. It should be moist, and if you touch it, the flesh should bounce back. Gills of the fresh fish should be pink or red. If you are into Ayurveda and Yoga and know what your *dosha* is, consider the following recommendation: freshwater fish is best for *pitta* and *kapha doshas*, while *vata dosha* does well with either saltwater or freshwater fish.

4. Try not to fry your food
Instead, grill it, boil it, bake it, or steam it. There are several reasons why: oils, even very healthy ones, like olive oil or coconut oil, still become oxidized under very high temperatures and prolonged cooking times.

5. Cook at least three to four times per week
Eat your food freshly prepared, within one to two days, to avoid ingesting decomposed elements, which can become moldy and acidic. It is hard to prepare fresh food every day

or two, but I have mastered it, even though it did not happen overnight. The key is to cook small amounts, depending on how many people reside in your household of course.

6. Chew your food well

The digestive process starts in the mouth, so don't short-change yourself by gulping the food down too fast. When the meal is not chewed well, the food fragments are still too big. This results in worse digestion and less nutrients being absorbed. It also results in extra food for the bad bacteria in the colon, which leads to gas and indigestion.

7. Eat mindfully

Food can only be healthy to you if it is eaten calmly and in full awareness, not in front of TV or computer, and not with a book. This can be a hard one to teach your kids, but if you start early, they will thank you later. Be mindful of what you are eating and try to internalize your meal's positive energy.

Your raspberries and blackberries are living things, and they are mixing their energy with yours by becoming your food. In my studies, I have come across food meditation, and I thought it was a wonderful thing. You can really feel the positive impact of the healthy, organically grown food on your Cells. Besides, if you just spend some tranquil, mind-ful time chewing your food and tasting its flavors, you will automatically wind up rationing and eating smaller por-tions, since you don't have that much time for eating during your busy working day anyway.

8. Have a cup of warm-temperature boiled spring water every morning, right after awakening

This will flush and soothe the Digestive System. I guarantee that it will help to regularize your bowel movements. This is also an ancient Ayurvedic tradition, which I cannot live without.

9. Avoid toxic additives, colorants, and preservatives

The best way to do that is not to buy packaged, processed meals. Shop only for fresh fruits and vegetables, meat, fish, and whole grains, and of course, nuts, seeds, and spices. Nothing else. Period.

This means that you will be avoiding 95 percent of your supermarket!

Your body will thank you for this shopping approach since 80 percent of some six hundred thousand processed foods on the shelves of the supermarkets contain added sugar. Bad sugar calories lead to belly fat, food addictions, and fatty liver and contribute to stroke, cancer, and diabetes. So, shop smart.

10. Make sure you eat enough fiber

Fiber is a kind of carbohydrate, which does not get digested by our body.

Soluble fiber absorbs water, which makes you feel full and slows down the rate at which sugar is absorbed into your bloodstream. Insoluble fiber keeps wastes moving through your colon, ensuring good and regular bowel movements.

This is why I am a huge proponent of eating fresh fruits and vegetables as opposed to drinking juices made from these ingredients. Fruits and vegetable have tons of fiber, while juicing eliminates this fiber goodness. Besides, what was the point of that thousand-dollar dental work last month, if you are going to be drinking your food? As I have said before, you have fangs for a reason. Put them to work!

11. Drink less alcohol and caffeine

I say this with a "heavy heart" because I love coffee and wine big time. However, we must face the truth that there are many downsides to drinking too much of either on a regular basis. Firstly, coffee blocks receptors for adenosine, a calming neuromodulator, and drinking too much of it literally makes you "bounce off the walls." Coffee and alcohol also make most people prone to insomnia and jitteriness. Both coffee and alcohol also have diuretic properties—that is, they make you run to the bathroom for number one and as such cause dehydration when consumed in excess. Alcohol is an interesting beast. On the one hand, it disinhibits us, which is my boyfriend's favorite reason why I should drink it more often. On the other hand, alcohol slows down our motor and cognitive capacity. To put it simply, it makes us clumsy and stupid. Of course, many people will have a natural question: But what about all those Mediterranean folks who drink wine and are not obese and enjoy good longevity? I strongly believe that Mediterranean health has to do less with alcohol consumption and more with the vegetable-rich diet, slower pace of life, taking time to spend with the family and friends, and taking long walks after dinner.

In short, my solution: if you love coffee, feel free to drink one to two cups a day. If you love wine and have no health issues, you can drink a glass on the weekend or at social events. Those of you who cannot live without having a small glass of red with dinner have my blessing as well. The point is to make yourself feel content, not deprived of something you enjoy.

12. Eat less red meat

I am big on Ayurvedic principles of eating, and red meat is considered the type of food that is least favorable for any body type. It is difficult to digest and has a heavy stagnant energy to it. However, if you feel like you must eat red meat, buy from the companies that treat their livestock humanely and raise it grass-fed, without hormones or antibiotics. Also, try to buy kosher red meat, as the process ensures that the animal's blood was drained thoroughly out of the body, that all the blood-carrying organs were removed, and the meat was then soaked in salt for several hours to drain the rest of the remaining blood out of the tissues. If your super-markets do not carry USDA organic kosher meats, you will have to rely on "butcher's promise" in regard to whether the animals were fed organically grown food and whether they were raised without hormones and antibiotics.

13. Remove all zero percent fat foods from your shopping cart

This stuff tastes horrible! Your ID will not enjoy it, even if you are highly motivated by my Phone App.

Summary

What is healthy for your Cells will be fresh, simple, and colorful. It will be real food, which should be a pleasure to eat.

APPENDIX 3

Be Happy!

> *Do not dwell in the past, do not*
> *dream of the future, concentrate the*
> *mind on the present moment.*
>
> —BUDDHA

A s I have pointed out earlier, if you are not occupied with work, sleeping, jogging, or having sex, the thoughts of food can easily creep into your head. But if you fill your present being with a feel-good kind of emotion, there will be less biochemical need for a food doping. Skim through these pages for some useful tips on how to fill your mind with joy so that it will not crave food when it is not supposed to. Of course, I do not expect you to do all these things; however, pick something that resonates with you and stick with it.

1. Get a good night's sleep

Getting a good night's sleep is one of my favorite things to do, in order to lose weight more effortlessly. You should be getting eight hours of sound uninterrupted sleep in order to allow your brain and the rest of your body to heal and repair. If you are insomniac, a hormone called leptin, which is responsible for making you feel full, decreases. At the same time, insomniacs who are not getting enough sleep have an elevated level of ghrelin, a hormone that is responsible for increased appetite.

If you stay up late, get up early for work, and not getting your eight-hour sleep, you will feel hungrier throughout the day and will not feel full when you eat, which is sure to make you eat much more than you are supposed to. On top of that, sound sleep improves the function of your prefrontal cortex, the part of the brain that deals with analyzing your impulses and inhibiting them when appropriate. So, by not sleeping well, you are much more likely to act on impulse and make bad food choices.

A recent study showed that teenagers, who were getting less than eight hours of sleep per night, had an average BMI (body mass index) of almost 5 percent higher than their counterparts who were otherwise leading similar lifestyles but were getting eight hours of sleep.

2. Enjoy buddy time with your Diet Slave No More! app

Seeing and hearing that cute stomach character's face before bedtime will feel so nice! Your ID wants fun, and your SUPEREGO would love to check in with someone who truly cares about your natural weight loss. When you hear that familiar friendly stomach character's voice, you are sure to produce some very happy hormones (serotonin and dopamine), which means good emotions.

3. Get in touch with nature as much as possible

Spending as little as two to three days anywhere in peace and quiet, with nature, can be an amazing doping to your balance and creativity. Exposure to nature in a tranquil setting makes us release plenty of dopamine and endorphins, our bodies' own opiates, to make sure we bring our body back into balance with good emotions.

Think of all the fun-loving Mediterraneans—they go on vacations one month out of the year. I know we are a much harder working nation, but let's try to take well-deserved breaks once in a while. Vacation time is a release for your suppressed spirit. On a daily basis, you are constantly doing something that is mandatory: going to work, surviving traffic, cooking, doing your laundry, cleaning, and so on. Our emotional release requires something that is not obligatory, and a small break poses a perfect opportunity for that. So take a couple of days every now and then, as regularly as you can, to refill your energy from nature.

4. Make your meals appetizing and a pleasure to look at
Your food should be pleasant in appearance, and you should present it to yourself on a nice-looking plate, if possible.

5. Eat before going out
I know that this will sound weird to many people since food is often the very reason people go out.

So, let me clarify: I recommend eating fifteen to thirty minutes before going to

- movies,
- comedy clubs,
- bowling allies,
- theaters,

- concerts,
- performances,
- gallery openings, and
- sport events.

When you are full, you become immune to the ever-present social pressures to eat badly (this means eating bad food and stuffing yourselves mindlessly) in these various contexts. Having a nice meal at home will make you more likely to focus on the cultural venue itself.

6. Move your body somehow

When it comes to physical exercise, there are different strokes for different folks. Personally, I never liked the gym routine: weights, treadmill, and elliptical machines. My favorite exercise is yoga and walking after dinner. That is what's personally fulfilling for me. I may not have the body of Demi Moore (I am referring to an actress of my generation, millennial reader), but I feel very comfortable with myself and feel that I keep my body-home in a good shape.

If you love swimming and have a pool nearby—swim. If you like Pilates and have a gym nearby—knock yourself out. Finally, if you like jogging or anything else that makes you release those endorphins—body's own opiates—pursue it on a regular basis. Work your core and your muscles whichever way you please.

If nothing else, walking after dinner, a traditional European *passeggiata*, which won my heart when I was visiting Italy in the early '90s, will do wonders for your digestion and clearing your mind at the end of the day. Just do what you enjoy to do—your ID will love it!

7. If you go to sleep later than 10:00 p.m., build a third snack into your eating schedule

If you don't do this, you will be entering the STARVATION MODE after around 9:30 p.m., and we all know that this state gains you pounds.

Eat to live healthy. Eat like a happy baby that you were. Eat to your peace as an adult that you are.

About the Author

S vetlana Kogan, MD, practices holistic and integrative medicine at her clinic in New York City. A Cornell University graduate, she received a scholarship from the National Institute of Health for her achievements in diabetes research.

She is an active member of both the American Medical Association and the Hypnotherapists Union. She has authored numerous print and online articles, including her own magazine, and has appeared as a medical expert on national television.

A patient observer of life and an outside the box thinker, Dr. Kogan has pioneered her own vision of Mind-Body medicine, where the best of what Eastern and Western philosophies can offer, are applied towards patients' well-being and longevity. She has also developed a revolutionary Uberdoctor™

encounter, which allows her to communicate with patients around the world.

Dr. Kogan is a mom of two great kids and lives in NYC. She loves reading, languages, and gazing at the Hudson River.

Made in the USA
Columbia, SC
29 March 2020